Getting the Best Care

Rescue Your Loved One From The Healthcare Conveyor Belt

Have Less Stress as You Protect Your Loved One from Suffering

Margaret Fitzpatrick, M.S., R.N., C.R.N.A.

For information contact: URPOINT, LLC   URPOINTLLC.com

This book contains information from many sources and gathered from the author's personal experiences. It is published for general reference and is not intended to be a substitute for medical advice from your physician or advanced practice nurse. The publisher and author are not rendering any legal, psychological or medical advice. The publisher and author disclaim any personal liability for information presented herein.

Cover Design by Constellation Book Services
Interior Design by Nick Zelinger
Edited by Kristen Havens
Additional Editing by Andrea Cumbo-Floyd, Yvonne Mullins
and Samantha Paquin

Publisher's Cataloging-in-Publication data

Names: Fitzpatrick, Margaret Mary, author.
Title: Getting the best care: rescue your loved one from the healthcare conveyor belt / written by Margaret Fitzpatrick, M.S., R.N., C.R.N.A.
Description: Includes bibliographical references and index. | Homewood, IL : Urpoint, LLC, 2019.
Identifiers: LCCN: 2018910568 | ISBN: 978-0-9747002-1-2
Subjects: LCSH Aging. | Patient advocacy. | Frail elderly. | Caregivers. | Dementia–Patients–Care. | Alzheimer's disease–Patients–Home care. | Senile dementia–Patients–Home care. | Hospitals. | Hospital care. | Hospital patients. | BISAC HEALTH & FITNESS / Health Care Issues | FAMILY & RELATIONSHIPS / Eldercare | HEALTH & FITNESS / Diseases / Alzheimer's & Dementia
Classification: LCC R727.45 .F58 2019 | DDC 610–dc23

QUANTITY DISCOUNTS ARE AVAILABLE TO YOUR COMPANY, EDUCATIONAL ORGANIZATION, ASSOCIATION OR OTHER ORGANIZATION for reselling, educational purposes, subscription incentives, gifts or fundraising campaigns.

For more information, please contact the publisher at URPOINT, LLC
Homewood, IL 60430. (708) 365-9136
Info@URPOINTLLC.com or Margaret@GettingTheBestCare.com

Contents

Introduction

"You'll never have to go to the hospital unless you break a bone or have another baby!"

This was my promise to my ninety-year-old mother. We both laughed at the prospect of her having another baby. Babies were her specialty, having had sixteen children. But my pact with my mother was a serious one. We were sitting in the kitchen of her ranch-style townhome, which she purchased eight years earlier after the death of my father. Those years had given her an independence she had never experienced before, and she was clear she wanted to be in charge of her destiny.

Excessive healthcare victimizes many people in this country. It subjects our oldest and most vulnerable patients to tests, procedures and medications that have little or no value to their health. What is worse, many are having medical interventions that are harmful to them. Patients and family members need to take control of the healthcare process and to know that, as people become older and more frail, less is more.

Too often people lose a sense of autonomy as they age. The healthcare system, well-meaning family, and society, in general, frequently treat the very old as if they were children. My mother was all too aware of that and determined to avoid it. She knew that she didn't want the final years of her life spent in a series of doctor's appointments and hospitalizations.

In the following chapters, I will tell you stories about people I have cared for: family members, friends, and patients. These stories impacted me in my early career as a critical care nurse and even now as a nurse anesthetist. You will also read about the widespread problem of unnecessary treatments for older people. These unnecessary tests, surgeries, and medications can lead to physical complications and declining health for an older person. Too often, vulnerable people are swept up into the healthcare system that always has another test to do or medication to prescribe. I view this as the "healthcare conveyor belt."

In my past training, a common assignment was to create a care plan for a patient. Having been told the age and medical condition, we were to outline a plan for that patient's care. We were never encouraged to speak with the patient to determine what her individual goals were or to ask what was most important to her. The assumption was each complaint and symptom could have a test and every test a diagnosis and each diagnosis a treatment. Looking back, I can see how limited that approach is. Instead, we need to assist each person in achieving her priorities in life in the best possible health, while also maximizing benefits and reducing the burdens of our interventions.

The process of protecting autonomy starts with having honest conversations with the people involved. Whether this is for yourself or you are helping a loved one, keep other family members aware, and let the appropriate health-care providers know about the priorities. This is the question I will keep reminding you about, which should be answered in any situation involving a healthcare choice: "What is the goal?" For some, the goal will be to remain at home with family or to avoid being in a nursing home, even if only for physical therapy after surgery. Many people have a goal of limiting medications, or they want to be pain-free. Once you have a clear idea of the goal, making healthcare decisions becomes less confusing.

My mother's goals for the last part of her life were to protect her autonomy and be at home with people who loved her. She wanted to avoid interactions with doctors and hospitals. Knowing those goals made my job easier as her primary caregiver. Situations arose during the final years of her life that could have easily led to hospitalizations and complex interventions. But I knew her goals, so each new health complication did not present a conflict or stress about which actions to take. Mother had made her thoughts clear on how she wanted to live. It was my job to ensure those goals were respected.

Alma: A Remarkable Woman

My mother was a remarkable woman. She came from a modest, small-town background and read more books and traveled to more countries than most people ever will. And, she did all that while raising sixteen children. She lived to celebrate her ninety-ninth birthday, and we were all blessed to have had her in our lives for so long. I was especially lucky in that Mother lived with my family for the last four years of her life.

Even though she suffered a severe decrease in her short-term memory during those last six to eight years, she always knew us and enthusiastically engaged in conversation. Her love of music and delight in small children never waned. And, although her physical capabilities declined, the need to see herself as a person with autonomy and dignity never diminished.

Maintaining Autonomy

With that in mind, I made her the promise that we would never make her go to the hospital (except to treat a broken bone or to have a baby). I realize that, given my healthcare background, it was less frightening for me to make that promise than it might be for others. However, I was confident that I could be her advocate and could get her what she needed while remaining at home. But I also believe that, with some planning and a clear discussion of goals, many more families can help their elders achieve a peaceful and comfortable end to their lives, rather than an institutional death. And you can maximize the comfort and enjoyment of your loved one's final years, instead of spending that time on repeated hospitalizations. We need to view old age as a stage in life rather than a medical condition.

Hospitals exist to cure people; the goal of the doctors, nurses—indeed, of the entire system—is to restore health. It is no wonder that, at the end of life, patients can be made to suffer. The system is not designed to prioritize comfort in the final stages of life. It is set up to avoid death at nearly any cost. And, the cost can be quite high financially, and cause physical and emotional suffering.

Most of us would agree that hospitals are not the best places to spend the final days of life. Studies repeatedly show that more than 70% of us want to spend our final days at home.

However, only 25% of us actually do. And, I would like to expand that to include the thought that most of us want to spend our final days, weeks, months and years at home (or in our home setting, be that our actual home, the home of a loved one, or an assisted-living facility). Yet, too many older people are enduring endless doctor's appointments and repeated hospitalizations in the last years of their lives. This leads to the majority of the dying process happening in hospitals.

The hospice movement has made great strides in the past twenty years. The growth in care has gone from 700,000 patients in hospice care in 2000 to almost 1.4 million in 2015. But even with those advances, hospice and palliative care are not available to everyone. While most large, urban hospitals have some form of a palliative-care department, smaller community-based hospitals frequently do not. There is a shortage of trained palliative-care healthcare providers. One estimate is that there is a need for at least 6,000 more palliative-care providers than are currently in practice. With the growth in demand and a shortage of providers, patients and families need to be able to request the kind of care they need. It is with that in mind that I want you to be able to advocate for yourself or your loved one using the information in this book.

Avoiding Hospitals/Doctors/Medications

"Grandma fell!"

This was the shout I heard late one night. Katie, my twenty-year-old daughter, was home from college and heard the fall. Rushing to Mother's room, I found her next to her bed, but, as always, in good spirits. Katie and I helped her back into bed after being sure she was not in any pain, which could have indicated a broken bone. I realize that having an older loved one fall is very frightening, especially if you are not a healthcare professional. It is understandable that there is an automatic call to 911. But, before you pick up the phone,

I would encourage you to take a moment to assess the situation, if your goal is to avoid subjecting your loved one to what may be an unnecessary trip to the hospital.

If your loved one is crying out in pain and distress, you may need paramedics to come. Anytime someone falls, do not be in a hurry to have her get up if she is on the floor. Wait and look; check to see if there is any bleeding or obvious deformity to the arms or legs. Take a minute or two to help her calm down, if she is upset, and ask about pain. See Appendix 1 for information on a guide that may help you to make decisions in these situations. Ultimately, it is up to you how comfortable you feel in dealing with these issues at home.

As we talked to my mother after helping her get back in bed, it was clear she had a slight facial droop, which is a sign of a stroke. It would have been "reasonable" to call 911 and head to the hospital.

We did not.

Here is my reasoning: Mother was not in any pain. In fact, she was not in any distress at all, just annoyed to have "bothered" us so late at night. I know the scenario that would have played out had we called 911:

1. Paramedics would arrive, take vital signs, ask questions and start an I.V. In general, this would cause a lot of (well-meaning) confusion for a ninety-six-year-old woman in the middle of the night.

2. An ambulance ride to the hospital's emergency department, where she would face more questions and tests.

3. A computed tomography (CT) scan would be taken
   and, if it showed no bleeding in the brain, then doctors
   would possibly recommend a medication called tPA
   (Tissue Plasminogen Activator). It can be a miracle
   drug for stroke patients, if administered within hours
   of symptoms and can help to avoid disability and
   post-stroke complications. However, it also requires
   the patient be admitted to the hospital and opens
   her up to other complications, such as abnormal
   bleeding.

When considering all of that, I asked myself, *What is our goal?* In my heart, as a daughter, I wanted to run to that emergency department and tell them to restore my mother to her full health. I wanted to ask them to make sure we would have twenty more years enjoying her cheerful and loving personality. Stop time and stop the inevitable, would be my plea.

However, I knew that my mother's goal was to be at home in familiar surroundings with people who loved her. I also knew that there are few miracles, but many dangers await the very old who go into the hospital. And so, we all went to sleep and waited to see what the next day would bring.

If Mother had been younger, our approach might have been different. Keep in mind that she was ninety-six at this point and had been clear about how she wanted to live. Going to the hospital was not what she wanted, and I was determined to honor her wishes.

In the following days, it became clear that Mother was much weaker. Even using her walker, she could not stand and walk without a lot of assistance. We were fortunate in that Mother was a petite person. At five feet tall and barely 105 pounds, it was not difficult to give her physical assistance when needed.

But that did pose a new set of problems. Mother could no longer be left alone for long stretches of time. My husband frequently traveled for business, and my workdays often went past 10:00 p.m., and sometimes required me to be on-call overnight in the hospital. This meant that we needed in-home care.

Getting In-Home Care

There are many resources available offering advice on choosing in-home care, but it is a difficult process to find a provider of in-home care with whom you feel comfortable. Having strangers come into your home and do such personal care means you have to find the right people. And, much like finding the right spouse, it is a challenge.

Initially, we hired a group of three women to share the duties; they worked independently, not as a part of an agency. They were recommended by a friend of mine who had this same group care for her elderly father. Each of them was experienced in performing personal care, and they were confident in their skills. But, after several months, I felt they were taking over my home, gradually putting their preferences, on how to do things, as a priority over my requests. And, so we contacted a home-care agency for personal aides.

The benefit of hiring independent contract workers was that I could negotiate the terms directly with the women them-selves, rather than dealing with an agency. But, we discovered the disadvantages of this setup when conflicts occurred. The independent contractors began to disregard our instructions, and we felt a loss of privacy and control in our own home.

Working with an agency would give us the advantage of having an intermediary who could mediate any issues we had with the employees. We used Home Instead® because the support staff in our local office were exceptional. I was relieved to have the option to appeal to the agency to intervene if/when issues arose. You have to consider this if you need outside help with personal care. Do you want to be an employer and have all the responsibilities that come with that? Consider that you may be more comfortable with a go-between who will deal with paying salaries and taxes and scheduling, as well as any performance problems that may occur.

But, just having the agency handle those issues did not solve everything. We still had to try out an assortment of people to find the best fit for our family. It took several months of trying different workers. Most of the women the agency sent were fine, but, for one reason or another, they did not work out. When a new person started, I would sit with her and emphasize the things we felt were most important in caring for Mother. Many of these women were very hard workers, but some felt they could nap while on duty or take extended smoking breaks, leaving Mother unattended. I felt that it was important to have an atmosphere of trust, assuming the best of the people we had in our home. I suppose I was naïve in feeling that demonstrating trust would foster loyalty. I think, in the stress of the situation, I did not acknowledge how vulnerable Mother was when no family members were home. And, because Mother had short-term memory loss, we could not rely on her to report any workers' behaviors that may have concerned her.

If I were to do it over again, I would have installed a camera-monitoring system in the hall, between my mother's bedroom and the bathroom. This would not invade my mother's privacy, but it would have allowed me to check in via my work computer to see how the aides were treating her. I would have let the aides know that we had the security system in place. The goal would not be to "catch" their bad behavior, but rather to foster a sense of security for my husband and me when we were not there. One thing we did let the aides know was that we had a large extended family, all of whom had access to the house and were free to drop in anytime, unannounced. I encouraged my siblings to come as often as possible to visit Mother and check on how things seemed at home.

Finally, we were blessed with an exceptional healthcare worker, who came to us through Home Instead®. Joann had a great deal of professional experience in caring for older people, but she embodied so much more. Her compassion and humor filled my mother's days with laughter and comfort. She quickly became a well-loved member of our family. Frequently, we heard them laughing as Joann readied my mother for bed in the evenings. It was wonderful to know that Mother had a real friend as well as a caregiver. No amount of thanks would adequately show Joann how grateful my entire family was that she came into our lives.

Refusing Hospitalization with Atrial Fibrillation

We had three more years with Mother after her stroke. Her health was good, although we rarely went to the doctor. Again, this may seem strange, but we had started decreasing these interactions with what I call the "industrial healthcare system" many years earlier.

Years before she came to live with us when Mother was in her late eighties, she started to experience intermittent periods of shortness of breath. She had been to a doctor who ordered tests, but never determined a definitive diagnosis. She was given an oxygen tank to have at her home and, occasionally used it when she felt the need.

One afternoon, she called me because the feeling of being short of breath became particularly uncomfortable. She wanted to go see a doctor because the shortness of breath had frightened her. Because it was a Sunday, we went to the emergency department where I had worked several years earlier, and I knew and liked many of the people on staff. Shortly after our arrival, Mother was given an electrocardiogram (EKG). The diagnosis was new-onset atrial fibrillation. This is not an uncommon ailment as people age; it is a particular type of irregular heart rhythm and can cause shortness of breath. It also was accompanied by a degree of congestive heart failure (CHF). CHF is also common in elderly patients, and at eighty-nine-years-old, we had to admit that Mother might just be elderly! CHF can be caused by the heart beating in an inefficient manner and fluid building up in the lungs. This contributes to the person feeling short of breath.

I knew that the staff would automatically admit her to the hospital, as it is part of the protocol for most patients who are newly diagnosed with atrial fibrillation. I also knew Mother wanted no part of staying in the hospital. So, I explained to the bewildered ER doctor that Mother would not consent to hospital admission. She felt much better having been given a diuretic, which eased her breathing. Diuretics are a class of medication commonly given to people with CHF. Heart failure—causing excessive fluid to "back up" from the inefficient heart and into the lungs—caused shortness of breath. The diuretic helps to eliminate the extra fluid. Now that those symptoms had been controlled, Mother wanted to be in her own home and to be treated by her own doctor.

We planned to visit her primary doctor the next day to discuss appropriate treatment options. Before leaving the ER, we obtained a copy of her EKG, chest X-ray, and lab results.

Having all of that information with us would help to avoid delays and repeat testing when we met with her doctor.

Having the Right Doctor

When we saw her doctor, Vanessa Hagan, she gave us different treatment options. It is routine for patients with this type of irregular heartbeat to be put on anticoagulants (sometimes called blood thinners). A common one is warfarin, also known as Coumadin, which helps to prevent small clots from forming in the heart, which can cause a stroke. These medications can be a great treatment option for the right patients. But, I knew if she were on warfarin, Mother would need to have her blood tested as often as once a month to ensure that she was not in danger of internal bleeding. It would also put her at risk for serious bleeding complications if she fell because warfarin inhibits the ability of blood to clot. We opted not to have it prescribed. Dr. Hagan was fantastic because she respected Mother's right to self-determination. After careful consideration, Dr. Hagan prescribed other medications to help control the CHF and heart rate. This compassionate and intelligent doctor helped us many times throughout the years.

However, years later when Mother moved in with us, we needed to find a doctor who was geographically closer. We knew this new doctor would primarily be refilling prescriptions. Because we made only the yearly appointment, which was required to get prescription refills, the new doctor never really understood our approach. She tried to advise Mother to eat a healthier diet. Our philosophy was simply: Once you reach ninety years old, you can eat or drink anything you want at any time! My husband would say, "If Alma wants a Manhattan and a piece of chocolate cake three times a day, who are we to refuse?"

The new doctor also suggested blood tests and an orthopedic consultation to find out if Mother needed a hip replacement. We politely declined, because again, what was the goal of these suggestions? We knew what Mother's goals were: limited contact with doctors and hospitals and time with her family to enjoy as much of her life as she was going to have. So, when I say, "We politely declined," I am referring to my mother and me. I did not make the choices for her. Instead, I made sure that we were all following the plan she had set out years earlier.

Chapter 1 Key Points

If you are helping someone else, start the process of speaking with your loved one about her goals and values for this stage of her life. Use this opportunity to ask for the gift of guidance from your loved one and give her the gift of an opportunity to speak openly about her thoughts and wishes. You should do the same for your family members—if you are planning your own healthcare goals.

- Use the Eldercare.gov website, which is a resource for services if you need in-home care, and read the information on AARP.org about having paid caregivers in your home.

- The Medicare.gov website has a comparison tool to search for home care. (Medicare.gov/homehealthcompare)

- Consider taking precautions to help you to feel confident about your in-home care, such as installing a camera that you can access remotely, and let everyone involved know the cameras are there.

- Speak with your loved one's healthcare providers for help in assuring that her values will be honored and her wishes respected.

- Involve as many family members as possible in the process of understanding your own and your loved one's values and goals.

- See Appendix 2, regarding power of attorney and advance directives.

CHAPTER 2

How to Avoid the Healthcare Conveyor Belt

Individual Healthcare Goals

Asking, "What is the goal?" is the filter through which we should view all medical decisions. What is the overall goal for this person regarding healthcare decisions? The specific goals may be different for a twenty-year-old with a fractured pelvis than for an eighty-nine-year-old with a broken hip. And, not all eighty-nine-year-old people will have the same goals. One who lives independently and travels frequently may have different goals than an eighty-nine-year-old with dementia and congestive heart failure, who lives in a nursing home.

It is possible to avoid your own suffering or that of an aging parent and your family members by preventing unrealistic goals from driving the course of treatment. Even worse than unrealistic goals is when there are no specific goals. In these cases, it can seem that the healthcare system puts the patient on a conveyor belt and runs him through the system, blind to individual needs.

Healthcare goals cannot be generalized; they must be individual. And they should be the guiding force for physicians, as well as for family members who are advocating for the person. No medication, test or treatment should be agreed to unless it is to further the specific goals of the person. If the medical care is directed by what the patient has identified as her goals and values, then she will not be on the healthcare conveyor belt. She will be in control of the care because her values are driving the decisions.

The Slippery Slope of Healthcare as We Age

Medicine has made so many incredible advances; it can be easy to think that there is a way to avoid the unavoidable. Our lives on this earth are finite; each of us will come to the end of life at some point. Birth and death are perhaps the only two experiences that all people throughout time will share. While it is natural and perhaps healthy to want to postpone the end of life for as long as possible, there comes the point when delaying is futile and even harmful. Indeed, research tells us that increasing costs and adding advanced medical methods for people approaching the end of their lives do not improve care but can increase suffering. Instead of prolonging life, we prolong death and misery. Both the patient and his family members suffer this way.

Studies have repeatedly shown that more than 70% of us wish to die at home, and yet, only 20% to 30% of us do. Why is there such a disconnect? It is easier to see the reason when you look at the patterns most people follow as they age or as a chronic illness progresses. This is the slippery slope of healthcare, which we can see all around us.

As we age, new health problems often creep up on us. We start to manage high blood pressure, perhaps diabetes, and then a heart attack or stroke; also, kidney disease and congestive heart failure may be diagnosed. These are common scenarios. Undoubtedly, these issues need competent medical management, although some of the most effective ways to control these conditions involve lifestyle changes. It is clear that all too few of us are willing to put in the actual work of changing our diets and increasing our activities. As a result, we become frequent customers for our physicians, who work diligently to prescribe the appropriate medications, treatments, tests, and procedures to help improve our health.

It is easy to see how the slippery slope comes into play. Healthcare providers prescribe more medications and tests are ordered; soon, you are on the healthcare conveyor belt. The conveyor belt puts you through "standard" sets of care treatments rather than an individualized plan. This was the case when the ER doctor wanted to admit Mother after diagnosing her new onset atrial fibrillation.

At what point do we step in and say "no" to more medical interventions? I knew that Mother did not want to be in the hospital, and I was able to ensure that her goals were the driving force in the decisions. It can be difficult to know, right away, what to do when you are surprised by a new diagnosis, and you have not made a plan. Do you refuse the suggested treatment or intervention? That is a highly personal choice, but it needs to be a conscious choice. It should come from considering how we want to live the final years of our lives and from having discussions with our loved ones, as well as our doctors.

Some things to consider when you're deciding:

- How many medical problems do you or your loved one have?

- What is the likely outcome of further medical interventions?

- What possible burdens do these interventions carry, as compared to the chances of benefit?

An important consideration regardless of age, but especially as we get older, is when and how to intervene, medically. We have to have a goal in mind before a crisis event because it is much more difficult to stop intensive treatments while they're in progress, rather than just not implementing them in the first place. If in the course of a discussion about healthcare goals, you learn that your loved one had decided he does not want to be on a ventilator, that goal needs to be understood by all those involved. Otherwise, if there is a critical health event, you risk your loved one being placed on a ventilator with a breathing tube, which would be the exact thing he had said he did not want. This often happens when the doctors and nurses who are caring for a patient do not understand their patient's healthcare goals. At that point, discontinuing that intervention becomes an emotional and sometimes difficult situation because of disagreements in the family as to how to proceed.

By contrast, if your loved one's goals had been well communicated originally, he may have had the opportunity for a more peaceful death that honored his dignity because it respected his goals. Discuss your loved one's goals (not being on a ventilator, for example) with his doctor, and if he lives in a nursing home, the nursing home staff needs to know. (Later in the book, there is information about advance directives that can help you share this important information.)

It's Too Soon Until It's Too Late

It always seems too soon to have a conversation about how we want to live the last months, weeks, and days of our lives—until it is too late. Have the conversations and make plans before your medical problems become overwhelming. Have your healthcare goals in mind and on paper and share these goals with the people you love. If you are caring for a loved one, help that person set her goals by having a straightforward conversation.

It is easy to say, "Have the conversation," but many people feel uncomfortable with it or that it is a morbid subject. In reality, talking about the end of life is a gift you can give someone. If the conversation is regarding your goals, it is a gift to let your loved ones know what your preferences are so they are not left wondering if they did the right thing. If it is a conversation you need to have with a parent or other loved one about her choices, then that, too, is a gift. You can give them the gift of letting them remain in control of their lives, even at the end of life.

One of the best resources I have seen is the Prepare for Your Care program (PrepareForYourCare.org). It is a well-researched and user-friendly website that walks you through the steps of clarifying and understanding your loved one's goals. The professionals involved in creating the Prepare for Your Care program were led by dedicated palliative-care physicians who were determined to create a method for people to understand and communicate their values and goals. The website has information in many languages, and it is purposely written in an easily understood way. It also includes several short videos that show common scenarios of people going through the process of choosing a surrogate decision-maker, as well as identifying their healthcare wishes and how they want to live the last part of their lives.

Why We Cannot Wait for the Doctor to Start the Conversation

We place a great deal of responsibility on our doctors. But, in the area of end-of-life planning, they are frequently ill-prepared. Until very recently, there was no formal training for medical students regarding this issue. Even now, it is inadequate, considering that, at some point, 100% of a physician's patients will die.

It is interesting to note that, while a majority of primary care doctors have a positive view of patients creating a living will or another advance directive, fewer than 50% have one of their own. Doctors who do have an advance directive are more likely to discuss this issue with their patients. Advanced-care planning is an area in which patients and family members need to be self-sufficient; doctors may not have the time or the inclination to initiate these important discussions.

Unnecessary Suffering When We Do Not Know the Goals: Mary's Story

As a nurse anesthetist, I frequently review charts and speak with patients about their medical history before surgery, which is called "pre-op'ing the patient." I was working in a small community hospital, where it was not unusual to see elderly patients from nursing homes who did not have any family present. Very often, I saw the patients late in the evening in anticipation of their surgeries the next day.

One night while I was making rounds, I saw Mary, who was a frail ninety-two-year-old with a history of advanced dementia. In addition to her multiple medical problems, because of her bed-bound status, her arms and legs were stiffly bent and immobile. She had bedsores on her back and feet.

Mary was scheduled to have a gynecological procedure the next morning. She had been experiencing some frequent, minor vaginal bleeding, and the gynecologist scheduled her to have a dilatation and curettage (D&C). This is a common procedure for women who are experiencing unusual vaginal bleeding, after a miscarriage, for instance. But I have never seen it done on a patient of such advanced age. I completed the preoperative paperwork and was not able to speak to the patient because of her advanced dementia. Mary's daughter had already signed the surgical consent.

The next morning, before leaving the hospital, I met with the anesthesiologist assigned to the case and asked him how this surgery could be justified. Mary would be subject to the stress of general anesthesia, her fragile legs would need to be secured in such a way to allow the surgeon to do the procedure, and she would have postoperative pain and cramping. Her dementia made her vulnerable to delirium and a prolonged hospital stay, which could increase her suffering and hasten her death. His response was what I have heard so many times in the years that I have been practicing: "The surgeon knows the patient and family better, and we defer to the surgeon."

When I asked the surgeon about this case, he said that the primary care doctor requested the procedure and that the family insisted on surgery. The pattern becomes: the anesthesia team kicks responsibility to the surgeon, who passes it on to the primary care physician, who typically says that the family wants the intervention.

However, the family is often under the impression that the doctor's recommendation is the most important thing to consider. Medical practitioners have not empowered families with the knowledge that there are alternatives to the endless tests and procedures. Too often, families rely on the medical professionals to give their best advice. And too often, the fear of litigation or lack of time with patients and families influences the advice given. Many healthcare professionals feel that by suggesting every possible intervention (CT scans, blood tests, MRIs, surgeries, etc.), they are protecting themselves from lawsuits. We seem to have lost the ability to provide patients and families with personal guidance and counseling concerning healthcare decisions. At the same time, patients and families are too quick to surrender their judgment to the doctors, rather than taking the time to ask probing questions about less invasive alternatives.

Of course, both the family and the healthcare provider want a good outcome for the patient. Unfortunately, practical considerations and time constraints may prevent the best possible individualized care. It is understandable how primary care physicians let the discussion of personal goals fall by the wayside, even with their very elderly patients. Research shows that the average doctor's appointment is just thirteen to twenty-four minutes, and other sources confirm that fifteen minutes is all you can expect of the doctor's time.

There are many pressures on physicians who have so little time to devote to each patient. After doing a quick physical assessment, refilling prescriptions, and answering a couple of questions, there is not enough time to have a thoughtful conversation about how a patient wants to live out the last chapter of her life. This inadequate communication leads to testing and treatments that may make sense for a forty-year-old patient but not for an eighty-year-old one. It is up to each of us to set an agenda and clarify the goals of the people we love, and then share those goals with doctors and other healthcare professionals.

Had Mary's family considered that the minor bleeding was not causing any discomfort to this very elderly, frail woman? Had they been cautioned that being in the hospital was exposing her to many complications, including infections and increased disorientation? Would they have given consent to surgery if they knew that more interventions done to this vulnerable woman would likely cause her more pain and discomfort without any real promise of benefit? Mary's situation was an example of low-value care.

For this reason, each of us needs to develop and share a set of goals and priorities for our own healthcare. Once we have those goals set, we can use them as a way to prioritize care. In order for healthcare professionals to make appropriate goals for a patient, it must be after comprehensive conversations that outline the patient's priorities and preferences. Those goals should come from the patient and family because they have to reflect the patient's values and concerns.

Chapter 2 Key Points

- Know that understanding the goals comes from many conversations with your loved ones.

- Unless there is very advanced dementia, most older people can articulate their preferences—even if it is simply to say she does not want to be on a ventilator (breathing machine) or she wants to be at home. See Chapter 6.

- You may be surprised to hear that your loved one has been thinking about end-of-life issues, but not talking about it for fear of upsetting you.

- Have the conversation with your family members who will be involved in the decisions. Discuss how you want to see your loved one live during the final chapter of her life.

- Use the available resources such as:
  PrepareForYourCare.org
  TheConversationProject.org
  AARP.org
  GetPalliativeCare.org/resources/caregivers/

CHAPTER 3

The Consequences of Undefined Goals

I am an advocate for life; I believe we should do all we can to live the best, longest life possible. This is why I advocate advance-care planning. I cannot say how many times I have raced into action when hearing my pager going off simultaneously with the overhead announcement of a "code." This is the alarm sent out because a patient's heart or breathing has stopped functioning, as in a cardiac arrest.

This emergency call is sent throughout the hospital to assemble a team of specialists, such as pharmacists, respiratory therapists, and nurses trained in advanced life support. A nurse anesthetist or anesthesiologist is part of the team to insert a breathing tube and connect the patient to the ventilator. Each time I respond with as much urgency as the time before. But, it is heartbreaking to get to the hospital room to find crying family members in the hall and to see several staff members performing cardio-pulmonary resuscitation (CPR) on an elderly patient with multiple medical problems.

My role in assisting the team is to manage the airway. I am at the head of the bed, getting a report on the patient. While I am inserting a breathing tube, I always ask the patient's age.

More times than not, the person is older than seventy with multiple medical problems. And, in my experience, those patients do not do well. I see them often "coding" several more times in the hospital stay, causing the emergency teams to come running each time. This is painful for the families to witness, over and over. Even after a "successful" code, an older patient with many medical problems rarely leaves the hospital able to function as he did before he came in.

The Realities of Emergency Codes in the Hospital

There is a lot of research about the odds of surviving a "code." When asked, people vastly overestimate the chances of surviving a cardiac arrest in the hospital. At best, the overall survival rate is between 17% and 22%, but the actual realities—for patients over age seventy and with multiple medical problems—are much worse.

The older and sicker a person is, the less likely he will benefit from the "code" team doing CPR and shocking his heart. Even if we successfully restore the heartbeat and circulation, these older patients usually do not leave the hospital alive. Fewer than two in ten will survive that kind of traumatic event.

Those times when we are successful in restarting their hearts, patients will be sent to the intensive care unit (ICU) on a ventilator for days or weeks. The odds of survival vary greatly, depending on where you live. Some areas of the United States have survival rates near 20%, and in others, the chances are less than 3%. Research has shown that when patients are aware that the odds of recovery are slim, those patients opt for less invasive measures.

Wanting "Everything" Done: Mr. Johnson's Story

Unfortunately, most patients and their families are not aware of the dismal odds of recovery, and this results in prolonged suffering for both. A particular example of this was the case of Mr. Johnson. I responded to a code called for him in the ICU. He was an eighty-year-old man with advanced lung cancer and kidney failure, which required dialysis. He had been in the ICU for more than a week with no improvement in his condition, in spite of all the advanced medical resources used in his care.

When I saw him, Mr. Johnson was barely responsive, only reacting to painful stimuli. Additionally, he was in respiratory arrest. His breathing had become so labored that it no longer would support life. The respiratory therapist, Tom, told me that Mr. Johnson's family "wants everything done." So, I inserted the breathing tube, and Mr. Johnson's hands were put into restraints to ensure he would not pull out the tube that was attached to the ventilator. I went back to seeing some post-operative patients in the recovery room. But, the picture of that frail man in the end stages of a disease that was taking his life haunted me. I knew he would die with those wrist restraints on and the noise and confusion of the intensive care unit.

It pained me to hear: "The family wants everything done." That is such an imprecise expression. What does "everything done" really mean? Is that revealing the attitude that in declining complex medical treatments we want "nothing done"? This is a tragic misunderstanding. What did the family mean by asking for "everything"? It seems to me that this is usually a plea from the family to restore the patient back to health, and everything should be done to accomplish that goal. Perhaps it would have helped the family if a healthcare professional explained that Mr. Johnson was not going to be restored to health because of his end-stage kidney disease and advanced cancer, in addition to his age. He was nearing the end of his life.

Possibly, the most appropriate question we should ask the family at this point is: "How would Mr. Johnson want the final days or weeks of his life to go?" Could we have told them that "everything" may mean chest compressions that might break his ribs, that we would shock his heart, insert a breathing tube, attach a ventilator, and put wrist restraints on? And, even with all of that, there is a low probability of his leaving the hospital alive. Might those words have reshaped their request for "everything"?

We must help families redefine "everything" to mean "everything that will help my loved one and not burden him with more suffering because of likely futile attempts at pro-longing his life." Then, the energy of the doctors and nurses can be focused on relieving any distressing symptoms and maximizing the quality time Mr. Johnson could share with his family.

After admission to the hospital, Mr. Johnson's family could have benefited if they asked:

1. What are the odds that my father will recover from this illness? Here, the medical staff could have informed the family that at eighty years old, with both advanced lung cancer and kidney failure, it was unlikely Mr. Johnson would leave the hospital alive.

2. What is preventing his recovery? Again, the doctors and nurses could help the family understand how his end-stage illnesses, as well as his advanced age, mean that Mr. Johnson is nearing the end of his life.

3. If my father's heart or breathing stops, what can be done to help him? The medical team has the opportunity to explain that they would call an emergency code; then, start chest compressions and insert a breathing tube. They could explain that there is little-to-no chance that Mr. Johnson would recover from a code situation and leave the hospital alive.

4. What treatments would you recommend that would benefit him the most?

Hopefully, the staff would recommend a palliative-care and hospice consultation for Mr. Johnson to help the family understand their options for helping him at this stage of his life.

We failed to present the complete facts to Mr. Johnson's family, and he and they paid a steep price. So much more could have been done to prepare them all for the inevitability of what would occur. Actually, before this progression of his illness, Mr. Johnson should have been given the opportunity to make concrete decisions for his life and death. Mr. Johnson and his family should have had the opportunity to understand that declining aggressive treatments, such as artificial ventilation and interventions directed to curing his already terminal-stage disease, does not mean he would be abandoned to die. Palliative care in the hospice setting, focused on comfort measures and treating distressing symptoms, is a dynamic and patient-centered specialty. Indeed, many studies have shown that, when offered early in the disease process, palliative care not only relieves suffering, it also maximizes patient health and can extend life expectancy.

Questions to Ask When a Serious Illness is Diagnosed

After the diagnosis of a serious illness, the following are some questions to ask the healthcare provider at the earliest opportunity to get the best outcome:

1. **What is the most likely outcome of this illness?**

2. **What complicating factors does my loved one have that make this a serious diagnosis?** These factors might include very advanced age and other medical problems, such as a prior stroke, emphysema, kidney problems, heart problems, cancer or diabetes.

3. **If we pursue aggressive treatments, what are the usual side effects of these treatments, and how will they affect her?** Treatments may require surgery,

and side effects may include pain, nausea, the need for extensive rehabilitation, and other problems that may affect your loved one's quality of life.

4. **Is it possible to have a palliative-care advanced practice nurse or physician be a part of the care team as we pursue treatment?** Palliative care can ease the burden of receiving aggressive treatments.

What Is the Goal?

What was the goal in "coding" Mr. Johnson? If you asked the family at that moment, their goal would be to have their father live. In the fog of the emergency, the only thought is to not lose their loved one. If we asked the participating staff, they would say to resuscitate the patient, to restoring his vital signs successfully. But, what if we asked the patient? What would he say?

Naturally, we could not ask Mr. Johnson at that moment. Indeed, even at the start of his hospitalization, it was too late to ask him because he had been brought to the emergency room with mental status changes and confusion. That conversation needed to take place months earlier as his cancer progressed. But, hypothetically, if we could somehow get inside his head, I wonder what would Mr. Johnson have wanted at that moment? My family had a rare opportunity to get that perspective when my father-in-law had a cardiac arrest.

After the Code: Pat's Story

Pat was a retired sergeant with the Chicago Police Department. He had joined the department after serving in the army and marrying the love of his life, Judy. He had a long and colorful career as a patrolman in the turbulent 1960s and 1970s, and then he led a special investigative team of the Chicago PD's auto theft unit. He never lacked fascinating stories to share with friends and family. The tales he told were especially legendary to his grandchildren.

His stories were about arresting the "bad guys," but sometimes they took a twist. A story that kept the kids entertained was one he told about being in a foot chase down a dark alley. The bad guy turned to shoot at Pat who dove behind a garbage can, only to immediately abandon cover because he discovered a large rat had made its home there. Pat told the kids, "I would have rather been shot than attacked by that rat!" This story made us laugh because it stood in contrast to the tough image of this often-decorated lawman. He was a formidable and sometimes intimidating presence in the lives of the many people who loved him.

Pat and Judy lived a modest life; a policeman's salary in those early years meant having to work overtime and part-time jobs to make ends meet. Judy maintained a pristine home while contributing to the family coffers by doing secretarial work and banquet waitressing when their kids were in school. Having raised three children on the south side of Chicago, they rewarded themselves with retirement winters spent in Florida.

A product of his time, Pat seemed to sustain himself solely on cigarettes and coffee. As he aged, his health suffered from bouts of congestive heart failure and emphysema. In his seventies, he was dependent on using an oxygen tank much of the time.

One terrible day in 2015, Pat became increasingly short of breath. Judy decided to take him to his doctor, but Pat became unresponsive in the car. I cannot imagine the panic that came over Judy as she frantically negotiated traffic to get to the emergency room. They coded Pat in the ER, and, with his heart rhythm restored, he was taken to the ICU on a ventilator with a breathing tube inserted. There is a protocol that is sometimes used in these circumstances after a cardiac arrest if the patient does not wake up after the return of heart function. The patient is kept unconscious, and on a ventilator, his body temperature is then cooled to well below normal. This cooling process is done in an attempt to preserve brain function after the brain may have been damaged by lack of oxygen when the heart stopped. At this time, the process was to keep him in the cooled state for twelve to twenty-four hours and then to slowly re-warm him over the course of a day. Meanwhile, family in Chicago planned to go to Florida.

I spoke with Judy several times during the next few days as she tried to get her bearings. She was distraught over trying to manage all of the decisions. She knew Pat since she was nineteen and could not imagine life without him. But she also knew he would not want to be on a ventilator. I encouraged her to follow her heart and to talk with their children.

Just after my children, Peter and Katie, arrived in Florida, something unexpected happened, and Pat's condition stabilized. Pat was awake and was taken off the ventilator the second day that Peter and Katie were there. They had a wonderful chance to sit and talk with their grandparents. Both in their twenties, Peter and Katie were fortunate to have devoted grandparents who treasured them since the moment they were born.

But, characteristically, Pat was blunt in his instructions. He told everyone, unambiguously, that he did not ever want to be on a ventilator or receive CPR again. Pat and Judy both knew that, in spite of this unexpected turnaround, Pat's health at its foundation was not good. His heart and his lungs were in bad shape, and he did not expect to leave the hospital. This was a rare opportunity for Pat's family to hear what he wanted. Most people would think Pat had a successful resuscitation. But, he had a different perspective.

The grandchildren left Florida, grateful to have had that time to talk with Papa Pat, but they knew that he would have preferred not to have been resuscitated that first day in the ER. He was in pain, and the experience of being in the ICU on the ventilator traumatized him. He wanted reassurance that he would not experience it again. Pat's instructions were respected when he died in the hospital the following day with Judy at his side, as she had been since she was nineteen.

Before Pat's death, Judy had told me that she knew Pat would not want to be on a ventilator, but when confronted with the panic of the emergency that day, she was not sure what to do. Even though they had been dealing with Pat's serious medical problems for several years, they'd never really had a specific conversation about what she should do if he stopped breathing. She did not feel prepared for the situation. If they had used a tool like the Prepare for Your Care website to clarify Pat's values, it might have eased Judy's emotional burden. Doing that sort of preparation much earlier in the course of his illness would have allowed Judy the reassurance she needed and would have let Pat feel confident that he was going to have his wishes followed.

Adjusting Goals to Reality

Many families face what they see as impossible choices. They feel they are being asked to decide if their loved one will live or die. The reality is that age or disease makes that choice, in many cases. The patient or the family can take action by setting a goal for how to live for the remainder of life. Perhaps the goals could be adjusted if everyone concerned had the facts about the likely outcomes of aggressive interventions at the end of life.

If you have a cardiac arrest at home or elsewhere outside of a hospital, the chances of survival are slim. The numbers vary, but generally, the survival rate is from 8% to 13%. So, between 87 to 92 people out of 100 who receive CPR outside of a healthcare facility will not survive the experience.

Many people feel that if they are already in the hospital, their chances of surviving after CPR would be much higher. Watch any of the television series set in hospitals, and you will see the dramatic efforts to shock patients back to life. Actors shout, "Clear," as they place the defibrillator on the chest of the actor portraying the patient whose heart has stopped. Suddenly, the character, who, moments before was dead, comes to life, recovering consciousness and everyone lives happily ever after. Unfortunately, those portrayals may have caused the public to have an unrealistic view of what happens for most people who receive CPR in the hospital. Even experienced nurses I have spoken to overestimate the chances of survival for patients. Between 17% and 22% of patients in the hospital who receive CPR live to be discharged alive. Half of those discharged will suffer from some level of neurological disability. Some are released to go home, others require significant rehabilitation therapy to regain strength, and still, many others are discharged to long-term-care facilities on a ventilator and with a feeding tube.

The reality is starker for patients over age seventy with more than one medical problem. If you are in your seventies with more than one chronic health condition, the uncomfortable fact is that you have a shortened life expectancy. Even for people who do not have a cardiac arrest, for those older than seventy with multiple medical problems, there is a high likelihood that you will have five or more years of disability before your death. So, it makes practical sense to think through exactly how you want to live and die.

Cancer, stroke and kidney disease are particularly difficult complications that lower the rate of survival after a cardiac arrest for people older than age seventy. Approximately, eight out of ten patients in the hospital who receive CPR die without being discharged from the hospital; for the patient older than seventy years old with kidney disease, cancer, pneumonia, or a stroke, fewer than 2 in 100 will survive after CPR.

The older you are and the more health problems you have, the lower the odds are that CPR will be effective. If it is effective in keeping you alive, and you are over seventy with multiple medical problems, you will likely need long-term nursing care and, perhaps, a ventilator and a feeding tube. More than half of older patients who survive a cardiac arrest in the hospital will go to a nursing home or rehabilitation facility.

A common scenario I have seen for the few older patients that survive and get to be discharged from the hospital after a cardiac arrest is that they will remain reliant on a breathing tube. It will require a tracheotomy (This is when the breathing tube is put through a surgically made hole in the neck and into the airway, rather than in the mouth to the airway.). They need a feeding tube surgically inserted through the abdomen to allow for liquid feedings. The patient, who is now dependent on the ventilator to breathe and on the feeding tube for nutrition, then goes to a skilled nursing facility. Would you consider this to be a successful outcome? It is a personal choice, and these facts need to be known for a genuinely informed decision to be made.

Yes, there are those "miracle" patients, stories that tell of amazing recovery against all the odds. But, I am seeking to empower you with the facts as they stand for most people. If you are caring for the healthcare needs of a loved one of very advanced age or one with multiple medical problems, you should consider these facts before he goes to the hospital for any reason. Ideally, you will have discussed what his healthcare goals are to know what treatment is appropriate. In any case, I would encourage you to explore the idea of having a "do not resuscitate" (DNR) order written by the physician for any admission of a patient of very advanced age, especially for those with dementia or other serious medical problems. This will prevent the emergency code team from being called, CPR would not be started, and the heart would not be shocked.

Chapter 3 Key Points

- Be sure that everyone involved has a chance to understand the complex medical issues that may be involved. Do your loved ones and other family members know the facts about the odds of surviving a code in the hospital?

- Make sure you and other decision-makers are aware of all of the medical problems your loved one has and how those problems impact his chances of recovering from a code.

- Understand what it means when someone says he wants "Everything done." Question this phrase. You may even hear it from doctors or nurses. Remember that it is imprecise and doesn't really convey a true meaning. Of course, you want everything done that may restore your or your loved one's health. But, do you want every piece of technology used to try to buy extra days of life if it is at the expense of suffering?

CHAPTER 4

The Realities of a Critical Illness

"It is the ability to choose which makes us human."
— Madeleine L'Engle

So often we hear people saying that they do not want to "be in pain" during the last part of their lives. It is hard to imagine being frail and in pain at the end of life. Yet, too often in a desperate attempt to deny the reality of life's finite nature, suffering is exactly what we bring ourselves and our loved ones. With conscientious planning and compassionate conversations, we can be prepared with a better plan. We can prevent the frenzied, often useless emergency procedures at the end of a loved one's life. One way to avoid this process is to discuss a Do Not Resuscitate (DNR) order with your medical provider.

What Is a DNR?

A "Do Not Resuscitate" order is not a "do not treat" order. Anyone who has a DNR order is entitled to vigorous healthcare and to have all of his health conditions treated. A DNR is simply a doctor's order that says if the patient's heart stops beating in a manner that can support life, and breathing is not adequate to support life, then what used to be called "extraordinary measures" to resuscitate the patient will not be employed. In other words, an emergency code should not be called to bring the code team running to the room and start chest compressions or insert a breathing tube attached to a ventilator, and no one should attempt to shock the heart into a normal rhythm.

A DNR order is most commonly written in the hospital. However, you can have a DNR order for someone at home or in a nursing home or assisted-living facility. It just needs to be a properly written order by a medical provider in accordance with the laws of your state.

Even with a DNR in place, any patient with cancer is still able to have chemotherapy and radiation, if needed. Any patient with heart disease, kidney disease, diabetes, and any other condition can receive required medications and treatments for those conditions. A DNR order in no way implies "giving up." Rather, it acknowledges that the patient and his family understand that resuscitation will likely be ineffective and may prolong suffering without meaningfully extending life.

As mentioned earlier, an excellent resource for starting the conversations about DNR orders and other important issues is the Prepare For Your Care website (Prepareforyourcare.org). You will find written and video guides there about how to explore goals and values surrounding health issues. There are also advance directives that include DNR orders, which are valid in each state.

Resistance Takes Persistence

There may be resistance from unexpected places when you ask about a DNR order. All relevant family members should be made aware that this is being done to honor your wishes if it is for yourself or to honor the wishes of your loved one who you are assisting. When a DNR order is in effect, family disagreements and misunderstandings are not uncommon. But, if it meets the goals your loved one has established, it becomes your obligation to advocate for it and not allow others to interfere. You can request that a social worker or patient advocate meet with the objecting family members so that they can better understand what is involved.

An unexpected place that you may meet resistance is from the hospital staff. When my father was eighty-eight, he had a minor stroke. It was my father's preference to be admitted to a large teaching hospital. I informed the staff physician that my father had a DNR order at home and wanted it included in the hospital record. I was surprised when the physician scoffed and said, "Oh, we are not anywhere near that point."

Not anywhere near that point? My father was nearly ninety years old with high blood pressure, a previous heart attack, a recent stroke and was obese. But, his health condition was beside the point. The doctor was inappropriate in not acknowledging his patient's stated preference to have a DNR order. I knew that the odds were that my father would not have a cardiac arrest while in the hospital, but it was certainly a possibility, especially given his medical history. And, my role was to advocate for what my father wanted; I was not there to appease the doctor. Reluctantly, the doctor wrote the order on the chart after speaking with my father and being reassured.

The reaction the young physician had when he scoffed at my DNR request is not uncommon. Many physicians are not comfortable with the concept of discussing DNR status, so they avoid it. Therefore, you have to be an advocate for your loved one and be prepared to overcome obstacles. Doctors are in the business of saving lives; their education and training are focused on identifying the causes of and ways to defeat illness. And, I am grateful for their expertise.

But, there are times in most people's lives when comfort care is most appropriate, rather than aggressive medical interventions aimed at curing an often-incurable illness. And we may serve our loved ones better if we acknowledge that old age is a natural part of the human life cycle and not an illness that requires advanced technology and complex intervention.

Post-Traumatic Stress in the ICU

My father-in-law, Pat, had indicated that he did not want to have any resuscitation efforts again. That may be surprising until we look at the actual effects of critical illness and the long-term side effects of being in the ICU. There is more research now showing that many patients suffer from a form of post-traumatic stress disorder (PTSD) after having been critically ill in an intensive care unit.

This type of PTSD is called Post-Intensive Care Syndrome (PICS). Think about it for yourself; imagine you are conscious of being in a bed, attached to a ventilator that is controlling your breathing; your hands may be tied in restraints to prevent you from dislodging the breathing tube, and you may be receiving intravenous sedation. You have no control over the situation while strangers are physically manipulating your body as they care for your needs. There is no clear sense of daytime and nighttime as you drift in and out of awareness.

We like to think that the sedation is easing the fear and discomfort these circumstances can cause. I certainly believed that when I was a critical care nurse working in a busy surgical intensive care unit at a major medical center. I would respond with confident reassurance when family members were concerned about their loved ones who were sick and on ventilators. I pointed out the intravenous medications that were flowing into the patient's IV, letting the family know that we were increasing the medications for pain and sedation when we saw signs of distress in the patient. But, we are now learning that the very protocols we used to treat intensive-care patients may be causing them long-term damage. Indeed, heavy sedation for days at a time may be part of the problem that leads to the PTSD/PICS if the patient survives the hospitalization. Many continue to feel physical weakness and a sort of "brain fog" long after they have recovered from the illness.

The post-traumatic stress problems are not the only lasting effects of the ICU. Research has shown that, after discharge from a hospitalization that included an ICU stay, one-quarter to one-third of patients suffer from PTSD/PICS and one-third experience a decrease in intellectual functioning as compared to their pre-hospital abilities. This decline can include personality changes and depression, as well as difficulties with memory. These symptoms can look like the effects of a traumatic brain injury or Alzheimer's dementia and affect patients of all ages.

It seems that advances in medical technology have given us the false belief that they are all leading to improvements in patients' lives. While the exact causes of the PTSD/PICS and post-ICU mental decline are not understood, we have to realize that a hospital is not like a mechanic's garage. Though we can exchange body parts and even have mechanical devices take the place of our biological organs, very often a patient does not become "better than new" after treatment. We have not learned how to prevent damage to the brain that can be the result of the complex treatments we so vigorously employ.

New research has encouraged critical-care teams to change patient treatment in the ICU in an effort to avoid PICS/PTSD. These new practices are sometimes referred to as ICU Liberation. This research has led to the careful selection of sedation drugs tailored to the specific patient, as well as limiting the dose to just enough to help diminish the anxiety that patients may be experiencing. Additional emphasis is on managing pain effectively, as well as trying to get patients off ventilators as soon as possible. Guidelines that allow family members to participate in care and in getting the patient up and moving sooner are all parts of the new efforts in preventing the damaging aftereffects of critical illness. These efforts are relatively new in the area of ICU care, and while they do offer promise, many hospitals do not implement similar programs.

Unfortunately, the most fragile patients are the most susceptible to the complications of being in the ICU, and they have the least ability to return to their former level of functioning.

The burdens patients can suffer after an ICU stay should be part of the consideration when forming goals with your loved one. The research has shown that there are increased risks to patients who are older than seventy for psychiatric and cognitive complications after being admitted to an ICU. For a person who is non-verbal or on a ventilator, it is difficult to know how much suffering will be experienced.

When considering the age and medical history of your loved one, factor in:

- How age and medical problems will affect the odds that extraordinary measures will be successful.

- Investing more in excessive interventions and expense in the final months of life will cause suffering without extending life.

- Your loved one may have to cope with PTSD/PICS and/or a decline in cognitive abilities.

These are the considerations that I hope you will keep in mind when making choices about medical care. In my career, I have seen many families devastated by the reality that follows a "successful code." These families are often unprepared for their loved one to be in a long-term-care facility and dependent on a ventilator and feeding tube.

Alma's Emergency Surgery

The decisions you make will be personal and specific to what you and your loved one have set as priorities. And the goals need to be specific and need to change over the course of time. For Alma, it meant that having emergency surgery for a bleeding ulcer at the age of eighty-two made sense. At eighty-two, my mother was healthy with no chronic medical issues and living an active life in her own home. So, when she suffered a sudden episode of vomiting blood, we went to the emergency room.

The doctors tried conservative treatments, but after two days in the hospital, her bleeding reoccurred, and she needed emergency surgery after having a massive blood transfusion. If she were frail with multiple chronic medical problems, that surgery could have meant the beginning of the end. She would have likely suffered multiple complications with a prolonged hospital stay.

As it was, she did have a brief ICU stay and spent more than a week in the hospital. Even though she was an energetic and healthy person, her age slowed her long-term recovery. Her ability to concentrate, as well as her energy and appetite, did not return to normal for a full year. Had she had pre-existing dementia, respiratory, heart or kidney problems, those conditions would have likely progressed, and she would have been subjected to repeat hospital admissions that befall many older patients.

If she were obese or had other difficulties walking on her own, that would have likely contributed to a further decline in her ability to function and may have required admission to a rehabilitation or skilled nursing home. These are very common outcomes for older, frail patients after surgery.

Because of her prolonged recovery, Alma knew that she never wanted to have surgery again. She was aware that, although in good health, any subsequent surgeries would come with more risks of complications that would put her independence in jeopardy. Her priority, as she aged, was to remain as active as possible and remain in her own home.

It is About Much More Than a DNR Order

It's very critical that you understand that your loved one's goals are about more than just asking about a DNR order or being placed on a ventilator. Their goals are more about understanding someone's hopes and fears. But, it starts with a conversation. Talking about the end of life can be a challenging conversation to start. When is the best time? Who should be involved? These issues are unique to every family. But in general, if it is possible, having the conversation with more than one family member present may help avoid misunderstandings in the future.

One reason people find this subject so difficult to deal with is because we tend to think of it as a conversation about death. Let's reframe it to a conversation about life. How do we want to live? It is just that the part of life we are referring to is the last chapter of life, which can last many years.

There is no need to imagine looking at your aging parent over brunch and saying, "Dad, how do you want to die?" Thinking of it that way would make anyone hesitant. People over seventy-five years old are well aware that they have lived more years than they have ahead of them. You may be shocked to learn how much your loved one is thinking about his final days.

Many older people actually have anxiety and fears surrounding death that may be eased by talking. Anxieties about being a burden or being alone or in pain are common. All of these can be relieved by gaining a sense of control, by sharing thoughts and developing the plan. Doing this can help you and your loved one to have less stress and depression as you cope with the realities of old age.

Setting healthcare and lifestyle goals is essential to having a clear plan when things go wrong. Once an illness strikes, emotions and fear too often take over. You may find yourself with your loved one, in the emergency room, uncomfortable and upset. At that point, it is difficult to think clearly. Before you know it, you have gotten on the healthcare conveyor belt, and you don't know how to get off. It is difficult to get off the conveyor belt because there is always another test to do, always more doctors to consult.

In reality, if your loved one is over seventy-five, weak, and has multiple chronic medical problems, this particular hospitalization will probably not restore him to great health. In fact, he may not leave the hospital alive. That is not to say that the hospital caused his death. But, going to the hospital will perhaps not improve his overall health status and may even add to his suffering and discomfort.

Whatever you and your loved one set as goals, please be sure to let your physician know. Having the doctor on board for the plan will make life easier. Be up front about what plan you have and how you will need the doctor's help. Just having a living will is not enough. The doctor or hospital staff may not be aware of the plan or may not refer to it when needed.

The stories you read in this book illustrate the importance of helping your loved one to set healthcare goals. Without personal goals that reflect her values, your loved one is vulnerable to being put on the healthcare conveyor belt and experiencing suffering such as PTSD/PICS and mental decline that may not result in a longer or better life.

Chapter 4 Key Points

- If you have resistance from other family members, help them to understand the facts. Make them aware of the risks to your vulnerable, loved one of PTSD/PICS, as well as the facts about surviving a code.

- What are your goals for your loved one at the end of her life? Will she be at home, in a nursing home, or living with you? Are you primarily focused on making sure that she is not in pain, confused or frightened?

- Use a tool, such as the Prepare For Your Care website, to make discussions easier and to make an Advance Directive. I have never met anyone who regretted being prepared.

- What will your response be should her condition change? If these things are not thought about and discussed ahead of time, then when new symptoms come up, you may be inclined to call for an ambulance. Calling that ambulance sets in motion a whole series of events that can take the control away from you and what your loved one has set as her goals and preferences.

- Have a plan in place for how the goals will be communicated to healthcare professionals.

- Some older people may prefer to be in a hospital if the end of life is near. Do not assume that you know what your loved one's preference is; instead, take some time to have the discussion.

CHAPTER 5

Misinformed Consent: How the Informed-Consent Process Fails Us

If you have ever had a procedure or surgery of any kind, you have probably signed a paper giving your consent to treatment. This is known as "informed consent," because, as the name implies, you are entitled to have received information regarding the surgery and have the opportunity to ask questions. Ethical and legal guidelines demand that patients understand the risks as well as the benefits regarding the procedure.

Unfortunately, due to time pressures and other factors, the process is often not ideal. Patients and families can feel intimidated by the hospital setting and the unfamiliar language. This is especially true if there is an element of a language barrier between the healthcare provider and the patient. Even though hospitals have translating services available, I have seen doctors and nurses view it as an interruption or inconvenience, and so these services go unused. Even in the best of circumstances, there is usually not enough time or effort put into the process of getting truly informed consent for procedures and tests.

What Is Informed Consent?

This is a vital and necessary part of healthcare, and yet, too often it is treated as just paperwork. Without truly informed consent, patients cannot be active participants in the decision-making process.

The American Medical Association (AMA) explains informed consent as:

> "Informed consent to medical treatment is fundamental in both ethics and law. Patients have the right to receive information and ask questions about recommended treatments so that they can make well-considered decisions about care."

Those of us charged with the responsibility of getting informed consent will tell you that we carefully explain the risks of surgery or other procedures: bleeding, infection, disability, death, etc. In reality, a skilled medical professional can skew this process to suit her objectives. This is done unintentionally by not creating an atmosphere for real discussion. Instead, the doctor or nurse lists off a standard set of risks and hands the consent paper to the patient or family member to sign. This method often does not leave room for a conversation that is rooted in the patient's personal goals or values. I do not mean to sound cynical. Often, I know that this lack of real conversation around risks and benefits isn't conscious steering of the process. But, unfortunately, informed consent has evolved from a true method of educating patients into a defensive play on the part of some healthcare providers to avoid liability. We know that a procedure is scheduled, and the objective then becomes to get the signature on the dotted line so that the process can move forward without delay. There is so much pressure on hospital staff that efficiency can come at the cost of inadequate patient education.

Even when the informed consent process is done strictly "by the book," it is not enough. Instead of presenting the patient and family with a form to sign and a canned speech about risks and benefits, we should be starting with a conversation about the patient's goals. This is especially important for patients who are frail, dealing with multiple medical problems, or who are older. We have to ask what the patient hopes to achieve from the surgery, and what is the likelihood we will accomplish those goals?

Aside from surgery, there are diagnostic tests, CT scans, MRIs, blood tests and the like, which may not further your goals. Anyone who has been in the hospital can tell you that there is seemingly an unlimited number of tests. But, if you are helping a loved one with her healthcare decisions, I would encourage you to ask the question, "What will we do with the results of this test?"

If the test results will indicate if surgery is needed, and you know that surgery is not consistent with the goals, then there may not be a reason to do the testing. If the goals are to avoid hospitalizations, surgery, and further interventions, then giving consent to have many tests may not fit with the plan. Frequently, once a test is done and the results are in, patients get swept onto the healthcare conveyor belt that leads to ever-more interventions. When the end of life is approaching, whether it is in a year or a month, the more interventions that are done often cause more suffering and do not extend life.

The poignancy of the question, "What are your goals?" intensifies as life grows shorter. But, I would encourage you to use that as your opening thought whenever faced with a medical choice.

There Are Always More Tests We Can Do: Justin's Story

Although consent usually happens before surgery, there are times when you need to make choices and give consent during an ongoing surgery. I knew a family whose fifteen-year-old son, Justin, had suffered a cardiac arrest. We had successfully resuscitated him after prolonged CPR and having his heart shocked three or four times by the paramedics. After the initial days in the hospital, doctors determined the best course of action was to implant a cardiac defibrillator in his chest. These are miracle devices for someone who experiences sudden and what could be fatal heart-rhythm abnormalities. The small, implanted device senses when the heart has lost its rhythm and shocks it, with the goal that the heart's natural pacemaker will kick in at that point. Justin's parents spoke to the cardiac surgeon and consented to the surgery—typically, a fairly minor procedure.

During the surgery, the cardiac surgeon sent one of the operating room nurses to obtain consent for an additional procedure. The surgeon wanted permission to take a biopsy of Justin's heart muscle. In certain circumstances, a muscle biopsy may reveal the cause of the heart arrhythmia. But, was this informed consent? Was this an opportunity to discuss risks and benefits?

The surgeon was in the operating room with their son, and the parents did not have the opportunity to ask him questions. It was natural in such a stressful situation to assume that this biopsy must be necessary, and so the parents signed the consent form. Unfortunately, because of the biopsy, Justin started to bleed. The bleeding made it necessary to stop the procedure and delayed implanting the defibrillator. It was done without complications on another day and has successfully operated ever since.

But that experience is a lesson. There is always another test to be done, but should they always be done? We, in the healthcare profession, always want additional data. But that data may not change the course of treatment or further the patient's goals. And so, I encourage people always to ask how the test will impact the treatments that are already underway. Will the information from the test or biopsy substantially change our decisions?

In Justin's case, the answer was "no." The type of biopsy at that time was not helpful in diagnosing a cause for the rhythm problem he experienced. But, his parents did not have that information when they gave consent.

Many Tests and Procedures Do Not Benefit Older People

It is important to be able to trust your medical provider. But that trust shouldn't be blind faith because research shows the care we receive is often not consistent with best practices.

Best medical practices are those treatments that are proven to be the most effective with the least chance of harm. It seems simple to expect that your loved one's care would be guided by what has been determined to be the most effective and least harmful, but that is often not the case. In 2014, a study of the care given to more than 1.3 million Medicare patients demonstrated that more than one in every four patients had received tests or procedures that are known to be of little or no value.

The study outlined twenty-six different tests and procedures, among them, was knee arthroscopy for osteoarthritis; routine preoperative testing for uncomplicated surgeries, such as cataract removal; and many types of cancer screenings for people older than the age of seventy-five. In one year alone, up to 40% of Medicare patients had one of the twenty-six unnecessary tests or procedures. Each test and procedure has its own risk of complications.

Many medical providers feel that patients expect to have medications, tests or treatments for every complaint or symptom. Providers claim they are trying to keep their patients happy. Others order treatments and tests of little value for fear of being sued if the patient has a complication or bad outcome. And, the financial gain is a motivating force for some.

Unfortunately, the reality is that many physicians are compensated by how many tests and procedures they perform. It is hard to imagine that monetary gain does not play a role in the occurrence of no-value or low-value care.

In order to comply with informed consent, providers should tell patients whether a suggested test or procedure is likely to be of no benefit—that the risk of complications comes with little possibility of gain. It is hard to imagine that someone with age-related arthritis would sign a consent to have a knee arthroscopy, if the surgeon informed her that multiple studies have shown that physical therapy can give as much benefit as surgery. People with stable and predictable chest pain are unaware that, when they consent to stent placement in their coronary artery to open a narrowed area, they agree to a procedure that carries risks without any evidence that it will have long-term benefits.

Too often, people think that having one of the low-value tests or procedures can't hurt and might even help. You may, in your efforts to help your loved one, be willing to try anything the doctors suggest. It is natural to think your doctor would not suggest a screening colonoscopy for your grandfather who is on dialysis, unless it was warranted or that your mother should have an electrocardiogram (EKG), chest x-ray, and blood tests before her cataract surgery if they are not needed. In reality, the colonoscopy to screen for cancer is not recommended for people older than age seventy-five unless there is a specific reason. And, a screening colonoscopy is discouraged for those on dialysis. The facts show that risks from having sedation, the chance of colon perforation, and the unpleasant preparation for a colonoscopy, are greater than any benefit the testing will have for an older person, especially one who has a life-limiting diagnosis such as kidney failure.

Similarly, having tests before low-risk surgery, like cataract removal, has been proven to cause more trouble than any benefit. *Even though the preoperative tests themselves may not pose a risk to older patients, it is the chasing for answers to explain abnormal results that poses a risk.* Just about everyone over age seventy will have some abnormal finding on one test or another. If the person shows no symptoms, looking for the causes of the abnormal finding may open a can of worms and lead to more testing. Meanwhile, they delay low-risk cataract surgery, while the healthcare team goes on a wild goose chase, trying to find answers to questions that no one was asking. The testing comes at a high financial cost, as well as putting the patient on the healthcare conveyor belt when all she wanted was to be able to see more clearly without cataracts.

It is up to each of us to decide what procedures, tests, and medications are in line with our goals. That is why knowing your loved one's goals and values regarding healthcare is so critical if you are helping with caregiving. It is unrealistic to expect our medical providers to tailor care to our needs if we do not have a clear view of our goals.

When Testing Does Not Meet the Patient's Goals

When Alma was ninety-eight, she needed to see her doctor to have her prescriptions refilled. It had been a year since we had been there, and most healthcare providers will not automatically renew prescriptions without a more recent physical evaluation of the patient.

Mother was not fond of these visits, even though they were infrequent. The hassle of getting there and trying to communicate with the doctor and staff annoyed her. Her lack of understanding was because most people did not speak clearly or loudly enough for her, although she wore two hearing aids. In addition, the providers and staff were usually looking at me when they spoke, so she did not get the visual cues one usually gets in conversation.

I have often seen this happen in my nursing career. If the patient is viewed as elderly, or in a wheelchair, or hard of hearing, doctors, nurses, and administrative people tend to direct everything toward the family member accompanying the patient. Imagine how this impacts the older person. If people routinely exclude you from the conversation, and it is difficult to hear them anyway, it is easy to "tune out" and ignore the situation. In my opinion, this can be a part of the mental decline in some people. If they are not engaged and a part of the process, could it lead them to shut down more? It is understandable because everyone is in a hurry. Time is short, and it is easy to fall behind on the schedule. Pressed for time, doctors, nurses, and others are looking for the fastest answer, and that may not come from a hard-of-hearing older patient. I tried to minimize this, and at the same time give a not-so-subtle hint to Mother's doctor by not answering the questions. I generally would repeat the question to Mother and wait for her to answer.

During this visit, the doctor said that since Alma was taking digoxin, a medication to stabilize her heart rhythm, she should get blood tests to make sure the digoxin was at an acceptable level. Mother asked what the test would reveal. The doctor explained that digoxin levels could be too low and, therefore, not effective, or it could be dangerously high. Mother looked at me and said, "No, I feel fine. I do not think I need a blood test." And so, we did not get the blood test.

Of course, if she had been younger, and not near the end of her life, I would have encouraged her to get the blood test, to see if a dose adjustment was advisable. Or, even if she were having distressing symptoms attributable to an incorrect dose, I might have encouraged her to get the test. But at ninety-eight, she did not want to have tests. She was comfortable with her decision to limit interactions with the healthcare industry, and I was there to support her.

Declining to have the blood test is a good example of how Alma was able to stick to her values and goals of limiting her medical interactions. She asked what the purpose of the test was and decided that she was comfortable with not getting the test. Although patients are frequently hesitant not to follow a doctor's suggestions, I know that it was easier for her to refuse the test because she knew I was there to support her decisions.

Lessons Learned as a Young Doctor: Informed Consent and Patient Goals

In his outstanding book, *Being Mortal: Medicine and What Matters in the End*, Dr. Atul Gawande recounts his experience as an intern in getting consent for spine surgery from a patient he called Joseph. Joseph had metastatic cancer and, at most, a few months left to live. The advanced cancer had caused a tumor to compress his spine. The spinal compression had caused some paralysis. The proposed surgery was extensive and complicated. At best, it would prevent further compression but could not reverse the paralysis that already occurred. At worst, it would expose Joseph to the risks of a lengthy surgery, anesthesia, and a prolonged recovery without the hope of an improved or a longer life. Because of his weakened immunity, Joseph was particularly vulnerable to postoperative infection and other complications. In spite of all this, he wanted the surgery. He did not want to have everyone "give up" on him.

Just the sentiment not to "give up" on him showed that Joseph did not fully understand the situation. The surgery could not cure or even slow the process causing his death, and it could not reverse his paralysis. Dr. Gawande recalled that Joseph was unrealistically seeking a miracle "at the risk of a prolonged and terrible death—which was precisely what he got." As a young, inexperienced surgery intern, Dr. Gawande did not have the authority or the expertise to sit and counsel this patient appropriately. I have seen interns put in this position because the more-knowledgeable attending physicians were very busy, but also because they simply did not want to deal with these emotionally messy discussions. Our doctors are excellent scientists and technicians, but many lack the skills or personal inclination to share difficult realities with patients honestly. Their training is to save lives.

Now, after years of experience, Dr. Gawande acknowledges that what would have benefited a patient in Joseph's position would have been to have a conversation asking what his goals were for his life and what he hoped to gain from the surgery. Asking Joseph what he meant when he said he did not want everyone to "give up" on him may have been a good place to start. Having a palliative-care professional on hand could have helped the discussion. Joseph needed to understand that the course of his disease was not going to be altered by the surgery and that he likely would spend his remaining weeks on a ventilator unable to communicate with his family. Indeed, the surgery, in all probability, would hasten his death. All of this needed to be communicated before asking for the consent to do the surgery.

In fact, I cannot see how a surgeon justifies doing this sort of surgery on a patient in Joseph's position. I was taught in my training that just because we can do something, does not mean we should do it. My view is that it was incumbent on the experienced professionals to help Joseph and his family understand that the surgery was not really a viable option. A more realistic, compassionate conversation with an experienced healthcare provider could have benefited Joseph and would have been a great learning experience for a young intern.

Similar scenarios play out every day in hospitals and nursing homes across this country, where patients are technically giving informed consent, and yet the process has gone astray. For patients and families, the best way to get informed consent may be to ask:

"Will the potential benefits of this treatment/surgery be greater than the likely burdens that it may cause me? I want to tell you what is most important to me at this stage of my life, and then you can help me to know if this treatment/surgery will fit into those priorities." Here, the patient and family can let the surgeon know that certain things—such as the importance of not having pain, or of not being on a ventilator or avoiding hospitalization—are priorities.

Will the Burden Outweigh the Benefit?: Gigi's Story

A consideration of whether a procedure, test, or medication has more burdens associated with it than it is likely to benefit the patient, is a crucial lens through which to view a medical decision for an older loved one. Unfortunately, this consideration is not in most informed consent discussions I have witnessed. One case stays with me because of this omission.

Gigi is a seventy-five-year-old woman with advanced lung cancer and emphysema, whom I met during her most recent hospitalization. Her condition has left her chronically short of breath and without appetite. It is common for people with emphysema to be seriously underweight. It is difficult to eat when you feel like you are suffocating.

Gigi is blessed with having a very dedicated long-term relationship with one of her doctors. It is obvious from what he writes in the chart that he is concerned for her.

She had developed multiple fractures in her spinal column, probably due to her advancing cancer. These fractures were causing extreme pain. Her physician, determined to find a way to alleviate the pain caused by the fractures, referred Gigi to an interventional radiology specialist. Interventional radiologists can perform a procedure called kyphoplasty on some patients with fractures in their vertebrae (bones in the back), and this procedure can do a lot to relieve pain for the right patients. The difficulty arose because, to do this procedure, Gigi has to be able to tolerate lying face down on the x-ray table for a prolonged period.

Weighing just eighty pounds and with limited strength, Gigi was lying on her stomach on the table in the radiology department when I was called to assist with the procedure. We needed to start a new IV line to continue, but her extremely depleted condition made it difficult. Cold and uncomfortable, Gigi endured multiple needle sticks to get the IV line and then discomfort from positioning her on the table. She was in pain the entire time; the physicians were hesitant to give her pain medications because of her unstable respiratory condition and low blood pressure. It was excruciating to watch her endure the preparation for the kyphoplasty on that X-ray table; I cannot imagine how she felt.

I do not know if Gigi and her family would have consented to the kyphoplasty had they known the extent of the discomfort she would endure. In theory, this procedure can provide a great deal of relief for patients at the end of life. Unfortunately, the nature of Gigi's fractures made it a long shot for it to be effective. This procedure is one that has been identified to be of little value to older patients. Would Gigi or her family have consented to go through with it had she been told that kyphoplasty was on a list of "low-value" procedures for some patients?

In any case, she and her family deserved to be fully informed of the suffering that she would endure while attempting to complete this procedure. And, a better plan could have been in place to make her as comfortable as possible while it was happening. Ideally, before sending Gigi for this procedure, her nurse would have verified that her IV was working. A forced-air warming blanket would have been available to maintain her body temperature, and a pain-management plan created before the procedure.

Most importantly, this particular procedure has been found to be of little help to patients like Gigi. Therefore, it would be more humane to offer palliative care instead of an expensive, painful, and, perhaps, useless intervention.

Questions to Ask Before Giving Consent

- What will happen if we do not do the procedure/test/surgery? Can it be delayed?

- Has this test (or procedure) been identified to be of low value to people like my loved one?

- How will the test results change the treatment plan? The answer gives you the opportunity to refuse tests when you know you will not consent to the proposed treatment.

- Will the benefits of this surgery, procedure, or treatment be lasting and more effective than the burdens it will bring after it's done? If the surgery, test or treatment has a low likelihood of benefiting your loved one but may increase her suffering, confusion or pain, you may want to reconsider.

- If this were your loved one, what would you do for her? This question gives you the chance to get a more personal response from the healthcare provider.

- How can you ensure that my loved one will be as comfortable as possible during this test or procedure? Will she be cold/confused/in pain?

Chapter 5 Key Points

- Informed consent should be a conversation when it involves a possible procedure or surgery for an older, frail person.

- Be sure that the healthcare providers know what your or your loved one's priorities and goals are and ask that they consider those as they formulate a plan of care.

- Be sure that you understand the possible complications that may come from any test, procedure or surgery, especially with your or your loved one's specific medical problems.

- Regarding any tests, you should ask: How will the results affect the plan for treatment?

CHAPTER 6

Advocating for a
Loved One with Dementia

Dementia is a term for many conditions that cause a significant decline in mental functions. Alzheimer's is the most common form of dementia and affects more than 5 million Americans. This is a heartbreaking disease that can steal away your loved one long before he dies.

The complexities of caring for someone with dementia can be overwhelming. Adding to the stress is the reality that caring for a loved one with dementia can make you, the caregiver, vulnerable to increased health problems and financial difficulties. It is vitally important that you plan for your own care, as well, during this stressful time.

There are many wonderful online resources that can help, including the Alzheimer's Association (ALZ.org) and the American Association of Retired Persons (AARP.org), in addition to social media support groups. Take advantage of the information these organizations have gathered; you do not have to go through this alone.

This is a disease that takes its toll on the entire family. Because dementia is a fatal and progressive illness, it is best to talk with your loved one early in the process to find out what she wants from her healthcare. Ideally, you will have had the conversation about how your loved one wants to live the final weeks, months and years of her life well before dementia prevents meaningful discussions. If you have not had this conversation, then the responsibility of setting the goals will fall on you. Having that additional responsibility adds to the stress of being a caregiver.

Having the Conversation Can Still Be Possible

In my experience, a dementia diagnosis frequently means that healthcare professionals will not consult the patient about decisions. This is unfortunate and not always necessary.

There are degrees of dementia, just as there are with other illnesses. Your loved one may not have the capacity to live alone or make complicated financial plans, but may be able to participate in a conversation about her healthcare choices and values. It is important to guard the dignity of the people we love, and part of that is to help them to be as much in charge of their lives as possible. To help someone with dementia be a part of these conversations, here are some tips:

- Pick a time of day that is best for her. Some people with dementia are at their clearest in the morning, but some are night owls. Be sure to choose a time that benefits your loved one the most.

- Limit distractions during the conversation. Perhaps small children or pets should not be in the room and have the television turned off. Tailor these situations to her particular preferences. If having a pet on her lap helps her think more clearly, then, by all means, make that possible.

- Sit with your loved one in a calm setting, and be sure to speak slowly and distinctly; take enough time to let her absorb what is being said.

- Be prepared to have the conversation more than once to ensure that you truly know what her feelings are about these issues.

The National Institute on Aging (NIA; nia.nih.gov) has suggestions for family members who are making healthcare decisions on behalf of a loved one. When you have not had the opportunity to have a specific conversation about what your loved one would want, they suggest using "substituted judgment." This is when you put yourself in the place of your loved one and ask yourself, "What would I want in this situation?" Another approach from the NIA is acting in the best interests of the loved one. Combining substituted judgment and best interests may help you to make these decisions.

Other Health Concerns

Dementia patients may have other health concerns that demand ongoing treatments. Diabetes, heart failure and kidney disease are common. Perhaps you and your loved one have decided to pursue more aggressive medical treatments during the early and moderate stages of dementia. He will continue his insulin and will check blood-sugar levels daily, or he will stay on his dialysis routine. These are common choices and are reasonable while your loved one is in the earlier stages of dementia. Staying in reasonably good physical health can help avoid hospitalizations, surgeries, and suffering that can accelerate the mental decline of people with dementia. In general, people live an average of four to eight years after the initial diagnosis of Alzheimer's. But, depending on an individual's health and other issues, he could live much longer with the disease. You need to have a defined set of goals and priorities as you are increasingly responsible for the care of someone with dementia.

As dementia progresses, your loved one's overall health will decline. The decline will mean that you will have more decisions to make. If the healthcare goals are clear to you early on in the process of caring for a loved one, then what others perceive as a medical crisis need not derail your plan. For example, if your loved one stops eating or drinking or you notice any further mental decline, you can understand that these are likely part of the natural progression of the disease and may not necessitate calling an ambulance.

Handling Finances

Another area of concern that is best handled early in the diagnosis of dementia is personal finances. It is essential that you have this conversation as soon as possible to prevent potential disaster. Consider setting up automatic payments from your loved one's checking account to ensure timely payment of utilities, insurance and the mortgage. A helpful guide to managing someone else's money can be found on the Consumer Financial Protection Bureau's website: Consumer-finance.gov. More information is in Appendix 2.

Remember that the capacity to make decisions is ever-changing in dementia. Especially early on, try not to take over areas that your loved one still remains capable of doing. You can have a supportive role in decision-making that assists rather than overrules.

A Victim of Excessive Healthcare: Daniel's Story

Some of the saddest examples of patients seeming to be put on the healthcare conveyor belt involve people with advanced dementia. Family can be overwhelmed with the daily challenges of caring for someone whose needs seem endless. In trusting that healthcare providers will know what is best, there can be a tendency to become passive observers once the person is a patient in the hospital. This leads to needless suffering for the patient and the family. Daniel is a striking example of someone who could have benefited from goal-directed care.

Daniel is ninety years old and lives in an assisted living facility. The facility sent him to the ER with reports of a bleeding ulcer and mental status changes. He has advanced dementia as well as non-Hodgkin's lymphoma (a type of blood cancer), high blood pressure and dangerously low platelets in his blood, which make him vulnerable to spontaneous bleeding, such as with his ulcer.

Daniel could not give us his medical history due to his dementia. His son is his power of attorney for healthcare decisions, but because of family and job responsibilities, he was unable to be with his father for much of the hospitalization.

The assisted-living facility sent Daniel to the ER after staff saw blood in his stool. Going to the ER set off a cascade of tests and consultations with different physicians. This is a ride on the healthcare conveyor belt that accomplished little. Daniel had been in the hospital for two weeks with little improvement; he continued to be anemic and at risk for bleeding.

These are the tests the physicians ordered:

- Two chest X-rays
- Three CT scans of his head
- Three MRI/MRAs of the brain
- Ultrasound of arms and legs
- Blood for testing throughout seven different days
- Five electrocardiograms (EKG) of the heart
- Echocardiogram (ultrasound of the heart)
- EEG (brain-wave reading)
- Ultrasound of the arteries in his neck

Daniel endured so much over those two weeks, including having a filter inserted in a blood vessel in his groin to prevent a blood clot from traveling from his leg to his heart or lung. During this hospitalization, Daniel's mental status worsened.

We know that hospitalizations for older and advanced-dementia patients can cause disorientation, and some studies point to an ongoing decline of functioning, even after the patient returns home. Confusion is an understandable reaction when you consider the vast number of strangers involved, thirty-seven by this count: Seven different doctors in four different specialties consulted on his case, sixteen different registered nurses took care of him with the help of fourteen different nursing assistants. All of these people were in and out of Daniel's room, each doing tasks a little differently and according to a schedule and priority, not set by Daniel.

Everything in the hospital environment was unfamiliar and possibly frightening or confusing. And, the hard fact is that none of this was likely to extend his life or improve its comfort or quality. Daniel's experience is a stark example of the healthcare excesses that inflicts confusion, pain and suffering onto the most vulnerable among us.

A solution to all of this excess will not come from medical professionals. The healthcare industry will not lead in this area; it will focus on a cure, even when logic tells us that there is no cure.
Doctors who are treating a patient with whom they have no relationship—as what frequently happens when a nursing home resident is in the ER—will see a list of symptoms. For each symptom, a test, treatment or medication is ordered.

No one in Daniel's case stopped to ask *what is the goal* in doing all these tests and procedures. Realistically, the solution for this excess will come one patient and one family at a time. We would better serve Daniel and his family with a frank and compassionate conversation that starts with: "What is your goal for this hospitalization?" By hearing the family members' goals, we could find out whether they have a realistic viewpoint of Daniel's health status.

If you find yourself in this situation, with a loved one admitted to the hospital with advanced dementia and an acute healthcare problem (such as a bleeding ulcer), here are some tips.

1. **For every test ordered, ask, "Why?"** For instance, "mental status changes" was the explanation for at least seven different tests for Daniel; it was the justification the physicians gave for the testing. In reality, the doctors knew the primary cause for his mental status: advanced dementia and that it is an expected progression of the disease for his mental status to decline. In addition to that explanation, his blood loss and chronic anemia added to a decline in mental function. If there is a reasonable understanding of what is causing the mental status changes, why order more tests? Why are his routine and comfort compromised to get answers to a question that need not be asked?

2. **Next ask, "What will we do with the results of the test?"** For example, if the brain scans showed bleeding, a mass in the brain, or signs of a stroke, what would be the next step? Would anyone recommend that a ninety-year-old advanced-dementia patient prone to abnormal bleeding have brain surgery? I would hope not. So, then what is the point of the testing? Why

subject him to the confusion and disruption of multiple trips to the radiology department and in and out of machines to get images when the information does not lead to his comfort or a longer, better life? The stark reality is that to have these tests Daniel was taken out of bed, put on an uncomfortable cart, wheeled through the hallways onto elevators to wait in a cold and sterile room until it was his turn for the X-ray, CT scan or MRI. During all of this testing, lasting two weeks, Daniel was probably confused, cold, thirsty and alone. What was the purpose of all of this? How did any of it benefit him, especially considering the limited time he has left in his life?

Suffering On The Healthcare Conveyer Belt

Daniel's story is a perfect example of putting the patient on the healthcare conveyor belt. Without advanced planning, the family may think that Daniel going to the ER is reasonable. Someone is bleeding, so he needs medical attention, right? Not necessarily. If Daniel's loved ones had made a plan to avoid trips to the hospital, they could instruct the nursing home to call them first to discuss any changes in his condition. Alerting the family first gives them the chance to ask questions to determine whether going to the hospital is necessary and if it would fit into their goals for the rest of Daniel's life. These questions could have helped them to decide:

1. **Is he in pain?** If so, can the pain be controlled where he is rather than the hospital?

2. **Are there any changes in his vital signs?** Someone losing large amounts of blood may have an increased heart rate and a lower blood pressure than before the blood loss.

3. **Are there changes in his behavior, or is he less awake than he normally is at this time of day?** An extreme change in behavior may cause concern. But, if the staff is simply noticing his behavior has been changing "lately" that is not necessarily an emergency.

4. **How much blood was seen?** If there are scant amounts of blood, or if it is something that happened once, perhaps referring Daniel to see the physician during regular hours is more appropriate than a trip to the ER.

If he is not in pain, what would be the goal of going to the hospital? If his family had determined that it was best to avoid hospitalizations, tests, and procedures, a small-to-moderate amount of blood in one diaper might not justify all of the burdens that Daniel will face by entering the hospital. Indeed, even if there was a large amount of blood, and it was a threat to his life, would the hospital be the best place for him? He is ninety years old and has multiple, progressive illnesses that will take his life. Do his loved ones want his life to end in his own bed, in familiar surroundings, or the hospital Intensive Care Unit after enduring multiple tests, procedures and interventions?

None of the interventions or testing for Daniel at that time had a reasonable chance of slowing or reversing the progression of the diseases that were afflicting him. His cancer and advanced dementia, as well as his advanced age, were following the expected course toward the end of his life. The only thing a hospital admission would do is expose him to more risks, increased confusion, and complications from hospital-acquired infections and additional procedures.

Chapter 6 Key Points

- Dementia is a progressive and terminal disease. Making plans and discussing your loved one's goals and values early in the diagnosis is important.

- People with dementia have a variable capacity to make decisions. It is an ever-changing situation; so give your loved one every opportunity to exercise her right to make decisions for as long as possible.

- What is most important to you and your loved one, regarding the progression of the illness? Is it comfort? Or, is it the length of life?

- For every test that is recommended, ask, why? Ask how the treatment plan will be changed, based on test results. Remember that you have the ability to decline any tests, procedures or surgeries that do not meet your loved one's healthcare goals.

- If your loved one is living in a nursing home, ask to be called before the decision is made to transfer her to the ER. See Chapter 10.

Questions to ask your healthcare provider, when dealing with dementia, include:

- How advanced is the dementia?

- Does your loved one have other life-limiting medical problems?

- If healthcare providers suggest a medical procedure or surgery, ask if your loved one is likely to heal or if the stress of the procedure is likely to cause further decline. See Chapter 7.

- Is she taking medications that may worsen her dementia? See Chapter 11.

- Can she benefit from having a palliative-care doctor or palliative-care advanced practice nurse? See Chapter 8.

Things to Consider Before Hospitalizing a Loved One with Dementia

Hospitals present unique problems for patients with dementia. Many times, family members feel that taking their loved one to the hospital will provide a safe environment, solve a new medical problem, and possibly provide a respite for the caregivers at home. Unfortunately, this is often not true.

People with dementia frequently will experience a decline in their overall health and their ability to function after a hospital stay. The decline may be due to the stress of the unfamiliar surroundings or for some other reasons. They are at risk for falls in an unfamiliar environment and can have anger and behavior problems from increasing confusion.

Unfortunately, rather than restoring a degree of health, going to the hospital for many frail, older people can lead them into a revolving door of more hospitalizations after complications develop. Twenty percent of patients who have Medicare come back to the hospital within a month of being discharged. Among people who need help with one or more self-care activities (eating, bathing, using the toilet, or getting dressed), 30% are readmitted within a month after being discharged from the hospital. All too often, the hospitalization accelerates the decline of physical and mental health, and this is especially true for people with dementia.

Recommendations about Feeding Tubes

In addition to the risks of declining mental-status function, being in the hospital opens the door to additional testing and treatments, which can cause problems to a frail person with dementia. It is common for patients in the advanced stages of dementia to be very thin. Eating is an activity that often loses its appeal; difficulty with swallowing is common, or they may not have the capability of feeding themselves. These patients are said to be malnourished, and so a feeding tube may be recommended. This can make sense to concerned family members. We associate good nutrition with improved health, so, people commonly give consent for the feeding tube. Sadly, this is liable to cause more problems than it actually solves. The potential problems begin with the procedure and continue for as long as the feeding tube is in place.

Even if your loved one comes into the hospital for another reason, doctors will want to order tests if they become concerned about weight loss. There may be a consultation with a gastroenterologist (GI doctor) who, in my experience, will order an endoscopy—a procedure that requires sedation.

The GI doctor will insert a camera down your loved one's throat to examine her esophagus, stomach, and upper intestine. The doctor will likely explain that the procedure is recommended to rule out any physical problems, such as cancer in the throat and stomach, which may be causing the weight loss. The sedation required for this procedure can cause many problems for frail, older patients; prolonged sedation and increased confusion following the procedure are common.

Because the endoscopy will probably not find a reversible cause for her weight loss, the doctor will insert the feeding tube. It is good to note that in recent years, referrals for feeding tubes for people with dementia have decreased. It is less common than it was in the 1990s in most communities. The reason is that it is well established that tube-feeding (when compared with careful hand-feeding) *will not improve health* for a patient with advanced dementia. Indeed, it can lead to nausea, infection, diarrhea, increased use of wrist restraints, and bedsores. Even though they are less common now, feeding tubes are still frequently used in patients, especially in large urban areas, such as New York, Chicago and Los Angeles. The advice you receive from the doctors is influenced by where you live, in spite of the experts' advice.

The American Society of Geriatrics recommends that people with advanced dementia do not get feeding tubes because evidence shows that tube-feedings are not a benefit to these patients.

Tube-feedings do not delay the progression of dementia, and there is evidence that people with advanced dementia do not receive nutritional benefits, either. The doctors who specialize in the care of older patients point out that eating problems, as well as pneumonia and fevers, represent a natural progression of dementia and indicate the person is getting closer to the end of life.

It may be reasonable to think that recommendations for medical procedures should not be determined by your location. However, statistics show that a person with dementia in California or Louisiana is ten times more likely to get a feeding tube than a similar patient in Portland, Oregon, or Madison, Wisconsin. Local practice influences healthcare providers' recommendations. This is something to keep in mind when faced with that choice.

Regardless of location, doctors must obtain consent before inserting a feeding tube. As we saw earlier, sometimes the "informed" part is left out of the whole "informed consent" process. I wonder if, when getting consent for the surgical procedure of inserting a feeding tube, anyone has told family members that having the tube may increase the chances of their loved one having her wrists restrained. Confused people often pull at foreign objects attached to them. Healthcare providers view this behavior as dangerous, and so restraints may be applied. Restraining someone means she cannot move freely, and that may contribute to getting bedsores. Combine limited mobility with the diarrhea that frequently accompanies tube-feedings, and you can see how skin breakdown becomes a problem. It turns out that what started as an effort to improve your loved one's health has increased her risk of being restrained and getting bedsores.

In addition to bedsores, people receiving tube-feedings are less likely to have the social moments that come with mealtimes. If careful hand-feeding is an option, the patient has the opportunity to interact with another person for an extended amount of time. It takes two minutes and no interaction with the patient to administer tube-feedings. Resorting to tube feedings means missing an opportunity that could encourage more human connections for the person with dementia. Recommending tube-feedings for a patient with dementia can be an example of how the healthcare system rarely treats these patients holistically, considering all of their needs rather than addressing a series of symptoms. When we recommend a treatment that may increase the burdens to the patient or rob him of part of his humanity, we do that person a great disservice.

Pressure Sores

I want to make a special note regarding pressure injuries, commonly known as bedsores. These are painful skin lesions that can be the cause of great suffering for a frail, older person. People in the later stages of dementia may not be able to walk, so they spend much of their time in bed or sitting in chairs. This type of constant pressure causes the tissues to break down, and the resulting sores can be as deep as the bone. These sores can lead to generalized infections and death.

The best thing for vulnerable people is to prevent a pressure injury, rather than trying to treat it after it occurs. The most commonly affected areas are the lower back, the shoulder blades, elbows, heels, and buttocks. For the most part, prevention means keeping your loved one's skin clean and dry and not having her be in any one position for more than two hours at a time. Even small changes in position, such as rearranging pillows so she can turn slightly to one side, can help avoid continuous pressure.

I often see patients with bedsores on the operating schedule for what is called a "debridement procedure." Surgeons may tell the family that the sore will not heal due to dead or infected tissue surrounding it, and that debridement will remove that tissue. What is usually not discussed is that, when a patient is so frail, she has a severely decreased ability to heal after such surgery.

Questions to Ask Before Surgery

Before you give consent for a loved one with advanced dementia to have surgery on a pressure injury or for any other reason, I encourage you to ask these questions:

1. **Given her condition, is it likely that she will heal from this surgery?** Frail people have a decreased ability to heal.

2. **Will the surgery cause her more pain than she is currently experiencing?** Most surgeries involve post-operative pain. Frequently, people with dementia do not have their pain treated because they are unable to ask for medication or staff may hesitate to give narcotics to a frail patient. There should be a specific plan in place for how the post-op pain will be treated.

3. **Is it likely that the surgery will bring enough long-term benefit to the patient to outweigh the**

immediate burden of the procedure? The burdens include the pain, confusion from being in the hospital and further decline because of the anesthesia required for surgery.

4. **How will this improve the time that she has left to live?** For many patients, the stress of surgery and hospitalization may increase suffering and shorten their lives. Consider whether remaining where she lives is a more thoughtful approach.

You can see how this scenario makes it clear that taking your loved one to the hospital can put her on the healthcare conveyor belt. The conveyor belt starts with entering the emergency department and continues along with more testing, which leads to more procedures. All of these things present risks to a frail person with dementia. These risks are why many experts are recommending that older patients with multiple medical problems are better off being cared for at home, rather than be exposed to the dangers they face in the hospital.

Palliative Care as an Option

Caring for someone with a complex medical problem like dementia can be daunting. Frightening new symptoms may appear, and many decisions are necessary. It is understandable that we turn to people and institutions that are supposed to be experts.

Unfortunately, hospitals, as they exist today, may not be the best place to turn for help for a loved one who has advanced dementia. Many families have found that the answer to these problems is palliative care. Doctors and nurse practitioners specializing in palliative care are skilled at helping patients and their families to better cope with complex illness. Palliative care can be an excellent addition to the care the patient is receiving now. And, you can still use your loved one's primary care doctor.

We can be so busy making decisions, and all the effort that is going into the decisions will not change the eventual outcome. Slow down and be with your loved one where she is because you will not be able to turn back time.

Chapter 7 Key Points

- Lower your stress of caring for a loved one with dementia by making use of the many resources] available to you. You should check ALZ.org and AARP.org for more information.

- Keep in mind that, even if your loved one with advanced dementia has a urinary tract infection (UTI), antibiotics may not be helpful, and they do not extend the lives of people in this frail condition. Discomfort and risks of adverse drug reactions may be the only result of treating your loved one's suspected UTIs with antibiotics. (See Chapter 8, A Note About Antibiotics.)

- Be aware that any hospitalization will risk making your loved one's dementia worse. You have to weigh the risk of further mental confusion against whatever benefit may result from a hospital stay.

- Ask to review the list of medications that your loved one is receiving in the hospital. There is a real danger that she will be given sedatives to keep her "calm" or anti-psychotic medications, which can cause further mental decline. (See Chapter 11.)

- Ask if a palliative-care specialist can see your loved one in the hospital. If one is not available, ask if there is a gerontologist or a nurse practitioner whose specialty is caring for older patients. (See Chapter 8.)

CHAPTER 8

Options for a Better Life: Palliative Care and Hospice

We have all seen the heart-wrenching commercials for animal charities: the trembling puppy lost on a cold rainy night or the injured, abused kitten. These sad images inspire people to donate tens of millions of dollars every year to animal relief organizations. People can be issued fines and even do jail time for knowingly inflicting pain on an animal. And yet, every day we allow the most vulnerable among us to experience pain and suffering in hospitals and nursing homes. The suffering caused by serious chronic illness may not be easily measured, but there are ways to ease the burdens that dementia, heart failure, cancer, and countless other afflictions can cause.

What Is Palliative Care?

Palliative care is a specialty in medicine that focuses on treating the distressing symptoms of serious illness. It is appropriate to have palliative care at any stage of a serious illness. The goals for this care include treating the physical symptoms that cause suffering and *helping patients and families deal with the stress of serious or chronic illness. Another priority is to assist the patient in living the best possible life. Palliative-care teams involve physicians, nurse practitioners, nurses, social workers, and, frequently, chaplains and volunteers. Patients receiving this holistic approach require fewer hospitalizations than those who do not receive palliative treatment.*

There are no restrictions regarding what other treatments patients can have while receiving palliative care. Someone with kidney disease, for example, can still receive dialysis, and a person with cancer can still get chemotherapy or radiation. Anyone with a serious chronic illness can receive benefits from palliative-care specialists. People with cancer, COPD, dementia, kidney disease, liver failure, heart failure, and chronic pain can all benefit from palliative care to help with symptoms, such as pain, fatigue, nausea, constipation, shortness of breath, and a lack of appetite while they are receiving the standard or aggressive treatments in the hope of curing or stabilizing their diseases. This approach is also helpful for loved ones of the patient; it can assist them with the stress that goes along with caring for someone with a serious illness.

How Is Hospice Different from Palliative Care?

Hospice care is a type of palliative care; hospice care is for patients who are thought to be at the end stages of their disease. It is for patients who are expected to have no more than six months to live, although many patients can extend that time. Due to the current Medicare and Medicaid insurance rules, patients receiving hospice care have restrictions from receiving the types of treatments focused on curing the disease. Comfort treatments are the mainstay of hospice care.

I am not going to specify which treatments are continued or discontinued in hospice care, because these guidelines are subject to change at any time. It would be most helpful for you to consult a hospice program in your area to get the most up-to-date information. In addition to local programs, you can get good information on AARP.org. Just search online for "AARP hospice information," and read the patient information from the National Hospice and Palliative Care Organization at Caringinfo.org.

In a society that values technology and innovation,
it is easy to understand how we over-invest in aggressive
treatments for loved ones, even when it can be clear
that the end of life is near.
Whether we are looking at a cancer patient undergoing
chemotherapy in his last month or the ninety-year-old patient
with advanced dementia having a feeding tube inserted,
we tend to think that we can buy extra moments of life with
more interventions. Even if that were true, and it often is not,

would extra days filled with nausea, pain, depression
and confusion be valuable or enjoyable?

A Longer Life with Palliative Care

Studies are showing that, for patients who are nearing the end of life, increased technology and expense results in a lower quality of life. Hospice/palliative care is more successful at the end of life than many traditional therapies. Patients who have the benefit of palliative care experience less depression and even live longer than patients who received only traditional care. Family members of palliative-care patients also receive the benefits, experiencing less stress, anxiety, and depression. This research makes sense when we consider how a long and difficult illness can affect the family unit. The experience of disruption to routines, as well as the helplessness loved ones feel when trying to help someone through a critical illness, can be overwhelming.

If family members play a key role in understanding and implementing the patient's goals, then some of the helplessness can be replaced by feeling useful and empowered. Instead of watching their loved one struggle with nausea, pain, and depression, family members can help to improve the life that remains by advocating for palliative care. This benefit occurs for both terminal patients and those who receive palliative care for a chronic illness indefinitely while pursuing other treatments.

When palliative care is received early on in the disease process, along with more aggressive treatments, some patients live *nearly three months longer* than those who receive the aggressive treatments alone. Given this, it would be logical to think that palliative care would become part of the standard for patients with any severe chronic illness. If the goal of medical treatment is to extend life, then this study supports palliative care as an effective way to do it.

Unfortunately, I know from my work as a hospice nurse that, all too often, referrals for palliative and hospice care come in the last days of a patient's life. For people coming into hospice care, nearly 41% are in the last two weeks of their lives. Delaying the referral means that patients and families will not get all the benefits of hospice. It is especially unfortunate because, well before having hospice care, these patients and families could have benefited from palliative care.

In my experience, this delay of hospice referral is due to many factors. Often the patient and family members are not fully aware of the benefits and services of hospice care, so they do not request it. Plus, the patient may be afraid that she will lose her current doctor. In addition to that, many physicians are reluctant to refer people in their care to hospice. The reasons for this may be more complex, having to do with an unwillingness to acknowledge that the patient is approaching the end of life. Additionally, many physicians are uncomfortable in discussing this very emotional subject with patients.

Healing is Not Always Curing

Dr. E. Wes Ely, a physician who has helped to bring attention to the phenomenon of post-traumatic stress for ICU patients, points out that *end-of-life healing does not always mean curing*. He shows in his practice that people can receive emotional healing by sharing honest, caring moments with one another that can bring purpose and also ease the fear of dying alone.

In an article he wrote, which was posted on CNN.com, Dr. Ely remembered a patient who asked about euthanasia. Although his medical ethics wouldn't allow Dr. Ely to cause his patient's death, his compassion led him to seek another way to help. He knew that the request for assisted suicide might stem from fear and loneliness. Those feelings of fear and loneliness may be alleviated if the patient had someone who could make a human connection with him at this pivotal time in life. As it turned out, the nurse who Dr. Ely enlisted to sit with his patient needed help, herself. And the conversations between the patient and the nurse helped them both to heal. The mutual empathy and connection each of them made showed Dr. Ely that the "best remedy for angst is human relationship and community."

It is unfortunate that the majority of dying is done in hospitals because hospitals seem to alienate the very people whom the patient needs most. We substitute doctors' and nurses' busy interventions for the attention and care of family and friends. Even though loved ones may be present, the atmosphere can create the feeling that they are minor actors playing bit roles as compared to the medical professionals at the hospital. Contrast this to how dying has been dealt with throughout human history when friends and family were attending to the needs of the dying person. As Allen Kellehear says in his book, *A Social History of Dying*, dying as a "shared social-interpersonal affair is becoming endangered" as we increasingly rely on institutions to handle the process.

It is understandable that we have a loved one in the ICU after a sudden accident or brief, unexpected illness where the days and weeks before were spent in a valiant fight for life. In those times, medical technology seems to be a miracle that gives us hope as we try to restore health. But, when our loved one's age and physical ailments logically indicate that life is coming to an end, perhaps there is a better way.

A Death Among Friends: Aunt Louise

My mother's sister, Louise, entered the convent before her twenty-first birthday. Her life was spent in community with other women as a Catholic nun. Louise was a delightful and lively person whose life did not take place in a sheltered cloister. She lived in service to people in some of the most disadvantaged areas of Indiana, California, Utah, Nevada, Kentucky and Arizona. Some of my best childhood memories are of visiting Aunt Louise with my mother and siblings. I always felt that she was living an adventurous life. But, it was the end of her life that impresses me most.

Louise was in her nineties when she moved back to the Mother House in Indiana. The Mother House was the epicenter for her order of nuns, and it was where the older nuns retired. That is where my mother, my two children, Peter and Katie, and I went to be with Louise as she lay dying.

You might imagine a dark, quiet place where elderly nuns sit quietly praying. But that is not the scene that greeted us. It was a large bright building with lively and happy women who greeted us as if we were their own much-loved family. Sister Claire hugged my mother and my son, Peter, and, taking

Katie's hand, escorted us to Louise's small room. It was there that we found Aunt Louise looking as if she were sleeping comfortably.

In one of the four chairs that had been arranged for us sat a petite woman, Sister Ruth. Sister Ruth told us that Louise was never left alone. For the past three days, the women took turns in four-hour shifts, sitting with my aunt. They explained that this was their long-held tradition; that none of them would ever be alone at the end of her life. They had lived in community with one another since their early years, and they would be there for each other in the end, too.

We spent the following twenty-four hours sitting with Louise and visiting with this group of remarkable women. They laughed and shared stories about their shared adventures as their paths crossed around the country at their various assignments. Having known one another for more than seventy years, there were plenty of stories.

We were all at her side when Aunt Louise died the following day.

This experience was the best example I have seen of a "good death." Louise was not only in the company of those who knew and loved her when she died, but they had also cared for her for several days and weeks before her death. It was a most moving example of the loving relationships of faithful friends.

Louise's death stands in sharp contrast to what is so often experienced in hospitals. Too often, families are stressed, the atmosphere is sterile, and the patient is alone much of the time.

The experience of the end of life in the hospital too often
is driven by the institution's rules and schedules instead of
by the family's or patient's values and goals. The important
moments at the end of life and the opportunities for loved ones
to support one another get lost because of the mechanics of
the medical systems. We have lost the humanity surrounding
the death of loved ones. This robs not only the dying person
of loving support, but also her family and friends, and leads
to increased depression in the grieving process.

As we celebrated a well-lived life, I joked with Aunt Louise's friends, asking them if I could join their Order when I am eighty years old. It seemed that being a part of such a community is a great way to ensure wonderful care at the end of life.

Obviously, this sort of situation is not possible for most of us. Even if we have a family, it can be difficult to have enough people around who can provide good physical care. This is where the early involvement of palliative-care specialists can help. Even before hospice is an appropriate choice, palliative care can help connect you to services that can help to ease the burdens of a life-limiting illness.

Spending More While Getting Less at the End of Life

Naturally, as we age, the effects of chronic illnesses can compound and lead to more and more interventions. If people fall into the common habit of being passive participants in their healthcare, riding the healthcare conveyor belt, it is understandable how someone can be in the ICU at age eighty, eighty-five, or ninety with a distraught family, and be unsure about how to proceed. If grandma's blood pressure suddenly drops when she is in the hospital following a stroke, she will probably be rushed to the intensive care unit. If the decrease in blood pressure causes her to lose consciousness, the ICU team will "call a code." And, as we discussed earlier, patients who are frail and over seventy years old who receive this code treatment in the hospital have a very slim chance of leaving the hospital alive. And, that chance becomes even more remote with advancing age.

Similar scenarios happen every day in hospitals across the country and cause so much suffering for the patient and family. At what point does the family now request these interventions be withdrawn for grandma? Additionally, the continuation of aggressive medical care can cause financial hardship and disputes within the family. The financial consequences are personal for families and have a widespread impact on the U.S. economy.

In 2014, Medicare spent just over $10,000 for each person it insures. That same year, for those who died, Medicare spent just over $34,000. We spend more than three times more on people who are in their last year of life; yet, rather than increasing the quality of their lives, we often cause more discomfort and pain.

It is clear that we disproportionately spend our money in the last year of life. Of course, it may feel wrong to look at this from a financial viewpoint. It is difficult to argue that any medical decision should be made strictly from a financial perspective. However, the fact is that generally, increased spending does *not* extend life for older people, but does prolong suffering. So, we are spending more money for a worse outcome, regarding the quality of life, at the very end of life.

Surely, this is not the goal for you or your loved one. The responsibility is on each of us to think through these facts and come to a deliberate conclusion as to how we want to live in the final chapter of life. Leaving it to chance can put you or your loved one on the healthcare conveyor belt and may lead to unnecessary anguish.

Suffering That Could Be Prevented: Janet's Story

Janet is seventy-six years old, lives in a nursing home and has had dementia for ten years; she does not recognize her children. Two previous strokes have left her unable to walk, and she is almost completely nonverbal. After years of smoking, she has severe chronic obstructive pulmonary disease (COPD), which causes difficulty breathing. Additionally, when she came to the hospital, she was diagnosed with a urinary tract infection (UTI) and mental status changes.

Within two days of coming to the hospital, she had a CT scan of her head (which showed no new findings), an MRI of the brain (again, no new findings), a scan of her kidneys to rule out kidney stones, and she was scheduled for a procedure to insert a feeding tube because she could no longer swallow adequately.

Because no one was able to advocate for any specific healthcare goals for Janet, the goal became treating each symptom or abnormal test result. There is no calculation to determine whether each test or procedure would prolong her suffering. There are several standard interventions ordered, unless, and until, her family members request hospice or, at least, some form of palliative care. It is most likely that Janet will get her feeding tube and go back to the nursing home until the next perceived health crisis. We know that nearly 20% of frail patients who receive Medicare will come back within a month of leaving the hospital, more than 30% return within three months. The revolving door of hospital discharge and readmission is not contributing to these vulnerable patients' comfort or sense of security. Indeed, Janet had been readmitted three weeks after discharge and again a month later.

If Janet were my loved one, I would want the following for her:

- Before coming to the hospital and before a crisis developed, I would ask for a consultation by a hospice or palliative-care specialist to see what services would benefit Janet. If her COPD caused her distress, palliative-care providers know how to treat the symptoms to ease the discomfort.

- Additionally, I would request that Janet not have tests for urinary tract infections, unless there was a specific symptom that indicates it a necessity. Nursing home residents are tested far too often, and frequently antibiotics are given even when the test is negative.

A Note About Antibiotics

Antibiotics are not harmless treatments; they are powerful drugs that can cause devastating side effects in a frail person.

One such side effect is clostridium difficile, known as "c. diff". C. diff causes debilitating diarrhea and can lead to a dangerous inflammation of the intestines. This is an example of how overtreating a suspected illness (a UTI, for example) can lead to a harmful outcome. Also, the increased use of antibiotics in long-term-care patients has caused an increase in drug-resistant bacteria. Drug resistance can mean that if your loved one needs antibiotics for a serious infection, those drugs will not be effective.

Palliative care can prevent the need for a trip to the hospital and could provide Janet with calm, comforting care in her familiar surroundings.

Chapter 8 Key Points

- Palliative care is a specialty in medicine that focuses on treating the distressing symptoms of serious illness. It is appropriate to have palliative care at any stage of a serious illness. If no one offers you palliative care, you can request it.

- There are no restrictions regarding what other treatments patients can have while receiving palliative care.

- Palliative care is always a part of hospice care. The difference is that hospice care is usually only appropriate when a physician has determined that the life expectancy is six months or less. Palliative care is appropriate at any stage of a serious illness, even while aggressive treatments are being used.

- Family members benefit from their loved one receiving good palliative care; it helps the family, as well as the patient, to deal with the stress of a complex illness.

- You should refer to AARP.org and GetPalliativeCare.org for more information.

CHAPTER 9

Things to Consider Before Going to the Hospital

While some hospitalizations are unavoidable, improved planning and outpatient follow-up would help patients, and their families avoid spending billions of dollars on unnecessary hospital stays. This waste is using limited government resources and contributes to personal bankruptcy for thousands of families.

This chapter gives you information to consider before you consent to admit your loved one to the hospital. I provide this information, assuming that you have access to a personal physician or another appropriate healthcare provider.

People eligible for Medicare generally have reasonable access to primary care doctors and advanced practice nurses (APN). A primary care provider is a vital resource if you are responsible for your loved one's care.

As previously discussed, frailty is an important considera-tion when making healthcare decisions with, or for, your loved one. Healthcare specialists use many different ways to calculate the level of a patient's frailty. Most calculations consider the following factors, and the more factors that apply, the higher the risk of frailty:

- The number of chronic medical problems: heart failure, COPD, kidney disease, cancer and dementia cause a higher risk for frailty.

- The amount of help the person needs to complete simple self-care tasks, such as eating, toileting and dressing.

- The inability to walk.

- Significant recent weight loss.

Frailty is a vulnerability to physical stress, such as sudden illness and chronic long-term conditions. If you see your loved one has many of these characteristics, you need to discuss—with her healthcare providers—her frailty and how it impacts her long-term health.

Common Complications for Frail, Older People in the Hospital

For frail, older people, being in the hospital can present a minefield of danger. Not only are they subject to risks of infection and increased confusion, but the way they are treated by the hospital staff and the effects of the medications they receive can seem inhumane. They are subjected to restraints confining them to bed and told to take medications that cause harmful side effects. While each patient is unique, some adverse events are common to all or most older people in the hospital. Being aware of these risks may help you to advocate for your loved one and avoid hospitalization or take steps to offset the risks while in the hospital.

Of course, hospitalization may be unavoidable, such as if your loved one breaks his hip and needs surgery. Hip fractures are a typical reason for admitting older patients. The perils of complications after a hip fracture make it a vulnerable time. We have all heard stories about an older person who was previously independent and now "going downhill" after breaking a hip and having surgery. Unfortunately, many treatments are done, and medications are given without consideration of the patient being of advanced age. Not considering age when treating a patient can lead to avoidable complications. If you have increased awareness of these issues, you may be able to prevent some of the problems.

Whenever it was necessary for my mother to go into the hospital after she was eighty years old, my siblings and I made sure that one of us was at her bedside nearly constantly while she was in the intensive care unit and for the days after surgery. Staying with someone in the hospital is a tremendous burden for families, especially when the adult children have to work and have children of their own. Our large extended family made it easier for us to schedule someone to always be with my mother at the hospital. If it is impossible for you to make similar arrangements, try to have a family member or friend at the bedside for the first twenty-four hours after any surgery. Having a familiar person with your loved one at night can help avoid confusion.

Please keep in mind that there are no minor surgeries for anyone older than the age of eighty. Even the most vigorous older person can be knocked off his game by the physical effects of a surgical procedure. The time immediately following an operation can be a tricky time for an older person. They may become confused in the unfamiliar environment and not able to speak up for themselves as they normally would. In my mother's situation, she had been living independently, driving, and taking care of her own affairs before emergency surgery for a bleeding ulcer. Even though she was as sharp as anyone in our family before surgery, after surgery, she did become confused and disoriented.

A family member or friend at the bedside can be sure that pain is treated and may be able to catch alarming symptoms, such as delirium or difficulty breathing, that busy nursing staff may miss. Having someone there to advocate for your loved one may help her avoid getting unnecessary sedation, which can lead to her becoming more confused.

Additionally, a familiar face at the bedside can be a calming influence. You may be able to avoid having your loved one's hands being restrained if she is pulling on IV lines or oxygen tubing. If her hands are restrained, your loved one may be more likely to develop delirium and its complications.

The Real Problem of Delirium

Delirium is a sudden state of confusion or change in mental state. In general, it is a temporary condition, but it can result in long-term problems for a patient. Restlessness, disorientation, and even hallucinations can be a part of delirium or, most commonly, the person may seem lethargic and slow to respond to questions. Some patients may have a mixed form of the condition that displays a combination of these symptoms at different times. Delirium is not just a concern for patients who are having surgery. Older patients, especially those with any level of dementia or with multiple medical problems, are at risk for developing delirium while in the hospital. It is common for delirium to be misdiagnosed; the most common type is Quiet Delirium without the agitation and hyperactivity symptoms. Up to 87% of patients over the age of sixty-five will have episodes while in the ICU. Plus, 50% of patients having hip or heart surgery experience delirium.

Since it can lead to severe complications and be a predictor of who dies in the hospital, any new episode of delirium while hospitalized should be treated as a serious event. An acute stroke or infection or other causes for the behavior changes have to be ruled out. It may not be necessary to have a CAT scan of the head to eliminate a stroke as the cause. A careful physical exam and review of the patient's history may be sufficient. But, blood tests may be needed to see if there is a new infection, severe anemia, or other problem that could cause delirium-like symptoms.

The signs of delirium, such as confusion, excitability or lethargy, may come and go throughout the day. You may have heard the term "sundowning," referring to people becoming confused in the evening. This can be a form of delirium. It is distressing for visitors to see this sudden change in their loved one, and it should be taken seriously. Prevention is most important in avoiding more complications.

Having delirium in the hospital makes your loved one more likely to have a longer hospital stay. Anything that prolongs a hospital stay increases the risks of getting an infection. However, things can be done to decrease the chances that your loved one will have delirium.

Preventing Delirium

- Review your loved one's medication list; see Chapter 11 for medications that can cause delirium and discuss this issue with his doctor.

- Does he drink alcohol every day? Alcohol withdrawal can cause delirium, so be sure that the doctor is aware of the amount of alcohol that your loved one usually consumes daily; it need not be a large amount for the withdrawal to affect him.

- Ask the staff about any activity restriction, and help your loved one move or stand as much as possible; most patients are allowed to get up and move to a chair with assistance even if there are limitations. Being mobile several times each day can help avoid delirium.

- Does he have his glasses and/or hearing aids? Are there batteries in the hearing aids? Not being able to see or hear is very disorienting and can add to the risk of delirium.

- It is helpful to think of ways to keep your loved one oriented about the correct day and time. Proper lighting during the day and a darkened room at night may help your loved one keep track of the passing of time and have less confusion.

- To avoid sleep disruption, ask your loved one's doctor if it is possible to for the staff to check vital signs only once during the night, or not at all if the patient is sleeping. This will depend on the patient's condition and illness, but it is worth exploring.

- Dehydration can cause delirium; while in the hospital, be sure that your loved one is getting enough fluids and is urinating.

- Ask if there is a geriatric specialist (gerontologist or advanced practice nurse) who can consult on your loved one's case while in the hospital. Having a specialist is especially important for patients over the age of eighty or those older than sixty-five who have many serious medical problems. Gerontologists are authorities in the care of older patients and are able to adapt care to your loved one's unique needs.

- If rehabilitation is needed, explore how it might be done at home, rather than in a rehab facility. Getting back home may help to reorient your loved one; arrangements for home rehabilitation need to be made well in advance of discharge from the hospital.

- Increased weakness is especially common for older people. Anyone who is on bed rest for three or more days will lose muscle strength. Ask about having a physical therapist evaluate your loved one before discharge to determine if she needs physical therapy to avoid injuries once she returns home.

Because older patients are vulnerable to confusion and new delirium while in the hospital, it is vital that the doctors and staff know who the main contact is other than the patient. Your loved one may enter the hospital alert and suddenly develop delirium; at that point, there has to be a family member or friend who has permission to receive medical information for the patient. Even if your loved one lives independently, when going into the hospital she should write down the names, and telephone numbers of the people whom she decides can speak to her physician and nurses, on her behalf, regarding her care. She needs to give permission because privacy regulations prevent hospital staff from giving even close relatives medical information without the patient's consent. If your loved one has a healthcare power of attorney, she can still designate other people with whom to share medical information. All of these names and phone numbers should be written down and given to the admitting nurse. It is a good idea to keep a copy in case the original is misplaced. Each time you visit the hospital, verify with the nurse on duty that the emergency contact information is easily available to them. This is information that your loved one can give in advance so that it will be available if there is a sudden hospitalization.

Delirium After Surgery

Surgery presents multiple threats to the welfare of older patients, including a decline in mental function. In this era of modern anesthesia, it is possible to do many surgeries without general anesthesia, and there is some evidence that it is beneficial for vulnerable older people to avoid it.

There are circumstances when general anesthesia is necessary, such as with most abdominal surgeries and for open-heart and lung procedures. Or, your loved one may have a condition, such as severe scoliosis or history of complex back surgery, that makes regional anesthesia difficult. Additionally, general anesthesia is always the backup plan should regional anesthesia be ineffective or if an emergency situation develops during surgery. See Chapter 11, which has a list of medications that may not be appropriate for older patients. You can then discuss the medication selection with the anesthesia provider before surgery.

Research shows that nearly 75% of older patients will experience episodes of confusion after surgery. Having post-operative delirium puts patients at a higher risk for an extended hospital stay and for being discharged to a long-term-care facility. If your loved one already has dementia or other serious medical problems, she is at higher risk of having post-surgical delirium.

It is reasonable to ask the anesthesia provider (nurse anesthetist or anesthesiologist) if your loved one can have surgery under regional anesthesia, instead of general anesthesia. Regional anesthesia affects only a specific part of the body, blocking pain sensation from the surgical site. In contrast, general anesthesia affects the entire body and brain, using the effects of anesthetic gases to cause a loss of consciousness.

People over age seventy commonly need hip and knee surgeries. Most of these surgeries can have regional anesthesia as an option. In my experience, when explaining the benefits of regional anesthesia to patients and family members, there can be a concern because the patient says he wants to be "put out." In other words, he does not want to be awake and aware of the surgery while it is happening. It is understandable that patients would have anxiety about being wide awake during the operation. It can be a frightening prospect. That fear may be relieved if you are clear about what is involved with regional anesthesia.

The vast majority of patients who can benefit from regional anesthesia are safely able to receive medications that help to sedate them. Basically, most of these people take a nap during surgery.

Even if patients are awake at times during the procedure, they are relaxed and calm and do not remember being awake after the effects of the sedation are gone. This is known as "twilight anesthesia." You can reassure your loved one and confirm with the anesthesia provider that if the patient becomes upset or uncomfortable during surgery, she will be given more medications, up to and including converting to general anesthesia. It is rarely necessary to change to general anesthesia because the medicines used to induce the twilight anesthesia are so effective.

There are special considerations for older patients, even if they can have regional anesthesia with twilight sedation. Sedation can be considered deep or light, and the difference may be significant for your loved one. There is evidence that older patients who receive the light sedation have a decreased rate of post-operative delirium. According to that research, fewer of the lightly sedated patients died one year after surgery, compared with those who had deep sedation. Fragile patients with multiple medical problems and who require help with activities of daily living, such as dressing and bathing, are especially vulnerable. These patients may do better if they receive light rather than deep sedation. The level of sedation given should be discussed carefully with the anesthesia provider. Let her know that you are concerned about post-operative delirium, and ask what strategies will be used to decrease the risks.

Alma's Surgery: An Attempt to Minimize Risks

When Alma was a robust ninety-four-year-old, she fell and broke her hip. She had been on her weekly mission of mercy, driving her very frail friend to church and out to lunch afterward. This is a scenario that so many people fear: an aging loved one who had been independent becomes disabled after breaking a hip and dying shortly after. Thankfully, that did not happen to Alma. But, it did take some vigilance on the part of my siblings and me to avoid some of the common difficulties.

In the emergency room that day, Alma was in excruciating pain, but the doctor on duty refused to treat her pain adequately. He was concerned that, at her advanced age, she would be at risk of depressed breathing or losing consciousness. It was infuriating for me to have to sit with Mother while she writhed in pain. I spoke with the nurse and the doctor, trying to convince them by telling them that I would stay with her and monitor her breathing. Still, the doctor would not relent. It was as if we were in a battle of wills, and rather than appropriately caring for his patient, he was determined to defeat me.

I was relieved when the nurse came in with a syringe because I assumed that she had finally gotten orders for more pain medication. But, instead, she told me it was lorazepam (Ativan), which is a sedative. She said the doctor felt that my

Mother was anxious. I refused the sedative on behalf of my mother and said that she was anxious because she was in terrible pain. Sedation is not an appropriate way to address pain in a patient of any age. And, the unnecessary sedation would have put her at risk for delirium while providing no pain relief, which is what she really needed.

After several hours, Mother was transferred to her hospital room. She had an experienced nurse who understood my request that Mother not be given a urinary catheter. Catheters often cause devastating urinary tract infections, which can lead to many complications in an older person. I requested that she be provided with and use a bedpan when needed. A bedpan is inconvenient and may even be painful with a broken hip, but the risks that a urinary catheter carry are worse than the problems of using a bedpan.

I am fortunate to have many siblings who were able to share the bedside vigil duties to ensure Mother would not be alone. Everyone in the family knew to ask about medication and to refuse any sedation. We were determined to do our best to prevent any delirium from setting in. Still, even with all of our efforts, Alma did experience some episodes of confusion.

Her periods of confusion made us more determined to get her home as quickly as possible after surgery. We arranged for her to have rehabilitation at home, and one of us stayed with her until we could arrange for in-home care. Even with all of our precautions to avoid delirium, Mother did have several weeks of personality changes after her hip surgery.

Mother had always dreaded the time when she would not be able to drive. Alma saw driving as independence, and it was something she didn't want to lose. When my siblings and I decided that, for her safety, Mother should no longer drive, She did not take it lying down. Prior to the hip fracture, she had a couple of incidents with the car that raised concern.

And, we were worried that it would be too easy for someone to see her out and about, follow her home and into her garage to assault or rob her. So, when she came home from the hospital, we told her that until the doctor cleared her to drive, we would take the keys.

This mild-mannered woman, who always thought the best of us, suddenly started to shout about conspiracy theories. Her usual upbeat personality became unpredictable that first couple of weeks back from the hospital. Thankfully, her pleasant demeanor returned as she recovered from surgery. But, it was frightening to see such a change in her. Mother's post-surgical delirium gave us the briefest glimpse into what families must confront when a loved one is stricken with dementia.

The delirium that Alma experienced shows that it can happen, even when all of the precautions are taken. I am convinced that Alma's delirium was brief because we were vigilant in preventing her from having sedation and in having family with her as much as possible. Also, we got her home as soon as we could in order for her to recover in familiar surroundings.

More Hazards: Pressure Sores

As discussed earlier, frail, older people admitted to the hospital develop pressure sores at an alarming rate. Within a week of being admitted to a hospital, 15% of older patients will have a bedsore. Consider this risk before you have your loved one admitted to the hospital. Frequently, bedsores start as redness of the skin on the back, elbows or heels. It is easy to think the redness was a minor issue. In reality, it reflects the damage that is deep in the tissues. This tissue damage can become severe and leads to the death of more than 60,000 people every year due to infections and other complications.

Many people think that pressure sores are a result of negligent care. Florence Nightingale, who is known as the founder of modern nursing, is quoted as saying, "If he (the patient) has a bedsore, it is generally not the fault of the disease, but of the nursing." Medicare and Medicaid penalize hospitals that have patients who develop serious pressure sores while in the hospital. It is an accepted theory that the vast majority of pressure sores can be prevented. The most important aspects of prevention are for healthcare providers to identify patients who are prone to getting these injuries and to formulate a prevention plan. The care plan should include keeping the skin clean, dry and intact and making sure that the patient is not in one position for more than two hours at a time.

If your loved one is frail and has limited mobility, there are things that you can do while she is in the hospital to minimize the risk of getting a bedsore. Be sure to ask the nurses about your loved one's risk for developing a pressure sore. Most hospitals require an assessment of every patient's risk. Also, ask what the plan is to prevent a sore. Healthcare providers do have good intentions concerning this issue, but the reality is that with increasing budget constraints and staff shortages, the physical care of patients can fall by the wayside. It is important that you tactfully let the hospital staff know that these things are a priority to you and that you will monitor the care your loved one receives. Of course, this must be done diplomatically to avoid resentment. It can be easier to correct a situation if you have not had previous unpleasant encounters with the staff responsible for the care of someone you love.

Maintaining a friendly relationship with the hospital staff is key to being able to achieve your goals for your loved one's healthcare. If you are staying at the bedside, be sure to emphasize that you are there to help. You want to reassure staff that your purpose isn't to oversee their work; rather you are there to make their days easier. Offer to step out of the room when nurses come in to do an assessment or change dressings, for instance. Giving them the space to do their important jobs shows them the respect they deserve. Of course, it never hurts to bring a tray of cookies or a fruit basket to convey your gratitude for their care.

Falls in the Hospital

Patients older than the age of seventy are at increased risk for falling while in the hospital, especially if there is a history of falling. Even if there was not a severe injury with the fall, patients who fall while in the hospital do worse on discharge than those who do not fall. So, it is very important to help your loved one avoid this danger while hospitalized.

Risks of falling may increase if your loved one:
- is confused/disoriented
- has had a prior stroke
- uses a cane or walker

- takes medications for seizures
- has anxiety
- has a history of falling

The problem of falling for older people in the hospital is another reason why it is a good idea to have a family member or friend at the bedside whenever possible. It is natural to think that a hospital full of healthcare professionals would have sufficient staff to monitor your loved one and prevent a fall. The reality is that, even if she can ring for help, a patient may have to wait thirty minutes before someone comes to help her to the bathroom. It is easy to understand that delays like that will leave a frail older patient vulnerable to falling as she tries to get to the washroom alone. Even if, as a family member or friend, you do not feel comfortable in providing physical assistance, you will be able to help staff be aware of when the patient needs assistance.

Deciding to Avoid Hospitalization

A foolproof way to avoid complications of hospitalization is to avoid going there altogether, if possible. Avoiding hospitalization for a frail, older person does not mean that you are "giving up" on living. Indeed, as we have seen here, the hospital is a stressful place for vulnerable older people and can hold real danger.

Being in the hospital means your loved one may be treated by multiple physicians, each with a different specialty, who will order tests, many of which are unnecessary or may cause further problems. As people age, there will be increasingly "abnormal" results with these tests. Each physician is then likely to want an intervention to correct the abnormality. Unfortunately, many of these interventions, which may be justified in a robust younger person, can cause a series of complications for frail patients over seventy years old.

Even though it is well known that older patients are vulnerable to complications, healthcare providers continue to encourage aggressive interventions, even when the person is near death. *Twenty-five percent of Medicare patients have surgery in the last three months of their lives.* Complications in the hospital make them more likely to spend considerable time in the ICU during extended hospitalizations and to be discharged to a nursing home rather than to their own homes. This reality is in stark contrast to what most identify as their goals of having a good quality of life and being independent.

Surgeons acknowledge the risks to frail, older patients having surgery, and yet there is a drive in the clinical setting that encourages more interventions rather than less-invasive alternatives. Keep this in mind when you are helping an older loved one with healthcare decisions. Doctors giving treatment options may not have her personal interests and goals as their primary concern. It is up to you to keep her goals at the forefront when discussing options with healthcare providers.

You'll need to tell the healthcare provider what your loved one's goals are at this stage in life and ask that those goals be the driving force for all recommendations. For instance, for my mother, I would have said: "Alma wants to be comfortable at home and avoid tests and procedures. With that in mind, what are your suggestions?" Asking that type of question can be a good method to keep the professionals aware that your loved one is an individual and not just a set of medical diagnoses.

One way to help doctors and nurses personalize the recommendations they give for your loved one is to ask, "If she were your mother with this health history, would you recommend this procedure?" or "If you were in her shoes, would you want this procedure at this stage of your life?" Even if the response is, "Yes, I would want the procedure," it does not need to override what you and your loved one have set as priorities.

Planning for Discharge from the Hospital

The time to think about discharge plans is the day you arrive at the hospital. It may seem premature to be thinking about what will happen after your loved one leaves the hospital, but it is not. Getting a call at noon telling you that Grandpa is ready for discharge can put you into a panic trying to make arrangements.

Most hospitals have discharge planners, and you may ask to meet with one to help make plans. It is important to do that well before the day of discharge. The discharge planner should be able to tell you how to get the medical equipment or supplies you may need to care for your loved one outside the hospital, for instance.

On the day of discharge, ask for any prescriptions. You may ask that the prescriptions be called in to your pharmacy so that you can pick them up on the way home, rather than having to wait while you are trying to get home. Doing this will also be the opportunity to catch any problems with the prescriptions, instead of discovering them when you are standing in line at the pharmacy late in the day. You should get a list of medications with detailed explanations.

Appealing a Discharge Decision

If you believe your loved one is being discharged from a hospital too soon, you have the right to an immediate review of your case. You may feel that your loved one's medical condition has not improved enough or that you are unable to care for her at home because of new health issues that have developed. The Beneficiary and Family Centered Care Quality Improvement Organization (BFCC-QIO) in your area will conduct a review. The hospital cannot force you to leave before the BFCC-QIO reaches a decision.

Before leaving the hospital, the staff is required to issue a pamphlet called, "An Important Message from Medicare about Your Rights." This contains information that can help you. Being well prepared for discharge will help avoid return trips to the hospital.

If the discharge is to a nursing home, you still have the right to appeal it. The next chapter (in this book) has information about placing your loved one in a long-term-care facility or a nursing home.

Chapter 9 Key Points

- Frail, older people are vulnerable to complications in the hospital, many of which can be avoided or reduced if someone is at the bedside as much as possible.

- Give your contact information and any advance directive to the doctor, as well as to the nurses on duty. Keep another copy at the bedside.

- There are no minor surgeries for an older person. Speak with the anesthesia provider about adjustments to the anesthesia plan to avoid sedatives and medications that increase the risk of confusion after surgery.

- Watch for any signs of delirium, and notify the doctors and nurses if you see new agitation, confusion, lethargy or a decrease in responsiveness.

- Activity helps to avoid delirium. Ask about getting your loved one up in a chair or doing some walking in the hallway.

- Be sure she has her glasses and hearing aids, if necessary.

- Start to plan for discharge on the day of admission. Remember that you can appeal the discharge order if you feel your loved one is not ready to be released.

- Refer to Appendix 1 for information on how to get a guide to making decisions about whether to go to the hospital, in the first place.

CHAPTER 10

Nursing Home Considerations

Older adults often go from the hospital to a nursing home for short-term rehabilitation or more permanent placement. Having a loved one in a nursing home can be challenging. There may be emotional burdens for making this decision. It is common for family members to feel they are abandoning their loved one, or they may resent other people in the family for not offering to move the loved one in with them. Whatever the circumstances, there are some important factors to consider when caring for a loved one who lives in a skilled nursing facility.

How to Choose

Finding a quality nursing home can feel impossible, but there are resources that you can access for information. Medicare has a website (Eldercare.gov) that offers information and compares skilled nursing facilities based on certain quality measures. Another great resource for helping your loved one with nursing home care is the AARP website,

AARP.org. Use the search box to look for nursing home information.

If your loved one is going to be in a nursing home, it is important to demonstrate your involvement to the staff. You can ask to meet with the nursing supervisor to get a feel for the quality of care. During the meeting, you can learn:

- What is the ratio of patient-care staff to residents?

- What is the staff turnover rate? Having long-term staff can indicate that it is a place that values employees, which is good for residents.

- What is the amount of overtime or double shifts that patient-care staff work? Working long hours or more than forty hours a week can mean that the facility is understaffed, and the staff is overworked.

- How many registered nurses are present during each shift?

- How often a doctor will see your loved one?

- Which medical specialists are available: dentist, podiatrist, physical therapist, etc.? Ask who refers your loved one for specialists' services.

- How does the facility provide hospice or palliative-care services? It is not unusual for hospice care to be a separate service you need to arrange for your loved one as a resident in a nursing home.

- Find out whether you can eat with your loved one on occasion. That will be a welcome treat for her, and it will allow you to sample the food and watch the staff interact with residents.

Important Things to Monitor

Most nursing-home residents require some help with one or more of the activities of daily living:

- eating
- bathing (washing body, hair and brushing teeth)
- dressing
- transferring (getting in and out of bed, chair and/or wheelchair)
- toileting

These activities take up quite a bit of the staff's time in any nursing facility. How these tasks are done is a major factor in the quality of care your loved one will receive. The physical care of residents allows staff the opportunity to have meaningful interactions with each individual. These tasks being done well also are a major factor in the health and well-being of the residents. The following section provides examples of things I have seen that demonstrate poor physical care.

Regrettably, over the past twenty years, I have noticed a decline in the quality of physical care given to the most vulnerable and needy patients. Whether it is because staff feel rushed and over-worked or the training is inadequate doesn't really matter. The fact is patients are suffering, as a result. There are things you can do to positively impact the care your loved one will receive.

Oral Care

One night, when I was on call in the hospital, I received an emergency page to respond to a code. The patient was newly admitted from a nursing home that evening with a fever and kidney failure. He now was unresponsive and not breathing. When I tried to put in a breathing tube, I found that debris blocked his airway. After removing the debris, I was able to place the breathing tube, but the patient died that night when the resuscitation efforts were unsuccessful. The debris that blocked his airway was a large crust of old food that had collected on the roof of his mouth over days or weeks and dried in place. At some point, that night it came loose and blocked his airway. The blockage prevented him from breathing and probably led to his cardiac arrest.

This story is a vivid indication of how not receiving careful physical care in the nursing home can lead to tragic consequences. In my experience, people who can feed themselves may have inadequate oral care. Your loved one's mobility may be limited, or she may not remember to brush her teeth or clean her dentures. If you know this is an issue, be sure to tell the staff supervisor that your loved one needs help in cleaning her mouth every day. Oral care is essential, even if your loved one does not have teeth or dentures. When you visit, try to notice how his teeth and mouth look. Pay attention to the condition of fingernails and feet also. If you notice that your loved one has dirty fingernails, it can be an indication of neglected physical care.

Skin Care

The skin on your loved one's hands and feet should not be dry and scaly. Dry skin can lead to developing open sores. Moisturizing his hands and feet can be a loving opportunity for connection when you visit. So often older people have lost a spouse and no longer have daily contact with their children, and compassionate touch is missing from their lives.

Research has shown that massage lowers anxiety and blood pressure. We know that infants need physical contact to thrive; it seems natural that older people also need that connection. Many of us can remember a time when we felt reassured by a comforting hug or an encouraging pat on the back. These are interactions that the frail, older person may not have, especially when living away from family. They may have daily physical care in that someone helps them to and from the bed, but that mechanical help is far different than a gentle hand massage.

In the years I spent working in a busy emergency room I cared for many people brought in from nursing homes. Each nursing home and assisted-living facility is different, of course. But I frequently noticed the patient's hands were dirty. All too often they had stool embedded under their fingernails. To me, this is an inexcusable lapse in physical care. In addition to just being a sign of neglect, it leaves the patient vulnerable to illness. It is hard to imagine ourselves eating with feces under our fingernails. Yet, this is something many vulnerable older people do every day. Dirty fingernails are easily cleaned with some care and attention.

If you do notice that his hands and feet need more attention, ask to speak to the nursing supervisor. It is standard to tell family members that staff cannot cut or trim toenails for fear of causing injuries that can lead to devastating infection. But, that does not prevent them from soaking hands or feet and trying to keep the patient's nails clean. It also does not prevent them from moisturizing the feet to help prevent cracked, dry skin. If toenails need care, request a podiatrist be brought in to see your loved one; this is something Medicare may cover, especially if your loved one has diabetes. The nursing home physician may need to write a referral for podiatry care.

Take an opportunity to speak with the nursing staff to ask about pressure sores and how the facility prevents them. If you can, check your loved one's heels, elbows and back for signs of redness or skin breakdown. If you see any indication that the skin is damaged, alert the staff and insist on knowing what interventions will be done to prevent further damage.

Preventing the Cycle of Rehospitalizations

It is important to know how often a physician or advanced practice nurse (APN) will see your loved one. Having these medical assessments may help to prevent trips to the hospital.

When nursing home residents go to the ER, it is usually outside of regular business hours: evenings, nights, weekends and holidays. This may be because the facility is short-staffed, or staff on hand are hesitant to wait until regular business hours for a medical assessment. These are sometimes thought of as "better safe than sorry" transfers. And yet, we have seen that being in the hospital can have harmful effects on the health of a frail person. Ask how often the nursing home sends patients to the emergency room and for what reasons. It may be unnecessary for residents to be disrupted by being taken to the hospital if a simple visit from the doctor or advanced practice nurse would be sufficient. If you are trying to avoid hospitalizations for your loved one, let the staff know and ask for an advanced warning before any decision is made to transfer your loved one. Having palliative care or hospice staff involved in your situation may be helpful for preventing trips to the ER. Frequently, these specially trained professionals will be able to treat pain, shortness of breath and other distressing symptoms that commonly lead to hospitalization.

Research has shown that more than half of emergency department visits by nursing home residents are preventable. Frequently, residents are sent to the ER as a matter of policy, after an injury or if there is a fever or unusually low blood pressure. But, not all such events are sufficiently serious enough to warrant a trip to the hospital or a designation as an "emergency." This is especially true if you and your loved one have a goal of avoiding admission to the hospital in the first place.

New symptoms, such as a fever, require staff to make a judgment call. When in doubt, most facilities will opt for sending a resident to the hospital. There is a fear that, if the staff chooses to treat the patient in place or wait and observe for further symptoms, they will be blamed for any complications. The sad reality is that skilled nursing facilities elect to transfer people to hospitals, even though these frail people are at high risk of having devastating complications in the hospital. Having an advance directive can be especially helpful in these circumstances.

Advance Directives in the Nursing Home

Everyone entering a nursing home or skilled-care facility is in a vulnerable state. Patients are vulnerable even if they are only there for a brief period of physical therapy and rehabilitation. It's wise to have an advance directive in place for anyone upon admission to a nursing home and anyone with a serious life-limiting illness or frailty when entering the hospital.

All too often, advance directives are written and forgotten. They are stashed in safe-deposit boxes or file cabinets with insurance papers and wills. Physicians, nurses, and other hospital and nursing home staff cannot honor someone's healthcare goals and values unless they know what they are. If you take the time to initiate advance directives, such as a power of attorney for healthcare (see Appendix 2), please be sure your family knows and that your healthcare providers are aware of it.

Another useful resource is the Prepare for Your Care initiative of the University of California at San Francisco. It is an easy-to-follow guide that will help you create an advance directive to share with your loved ones. An advance directive is appropriate for people at every stage of life and will help you and your loved one clarify your goals for healthcare.

If your loved one lives in a nursing home, there is another option for an advance directive. You or your loved one can request a "do not hospitalize" (DNH) order. Having a DNH will prevent the emergency calls for an ambulance should her status suddenly change.

After you request that the admitting doctor write a DNH order, you have to stay involved. DNH orders are most effective in slowing down the process of your loved one going to the hospital should there be a new problem. In actual practice, these DNH orders prompt the nursing home staff to call family or whoever is the designated decision maker concerning the possible hospitalization. Taking the opportunity to ask questions before an ambulance is called may fit more into the goals you and your loved one have established, rather than receiving a phone call that she is already on the way to the emergency department. Getting that advance call gives you the opportunity to intervene and ask that your loved one remains at the nursing home until you or another loved one can be present to evaluate the situation.

Medication Concerns in the Nursing Home

Ask to see a list of medications that your loved one will receive. Be sure that you periodically ask about medications and review any changes made to the list. In Chapter 11, you can see information about specific issues for older people and which medications to avoid if it's at all possible. Also, Appendix 3 has important information regarding recommended vaccinations for older adults. These vaccines can be especially helpful if your loved one lives in any kind of group environment.

Chapter 10 Key Points

- Carefully continue to monitor the care your loved one is receiving after you choose a nursing home or assisted-living facility.

- Mouth and skin care are particularly good reflections of the quality of physical care given.

- Be sure the staff understands any advance directive for your loved one, if you want to avoid hospitalizations, consider a Do Not Hospitalize order.

- Review medications periodically.

- See the Further Resources section at the back of this book for ideas of where to look for more information.

CHAPTER 11

Medication Issues as People Age

As we age, our bodies process medications differently. The way medications affect us is determined by many things. The percentage of body fat to lean muscle, and heart, liver, kidney, and brain function all influence how a medication will impact a particular person. As these things change over time, a drug that was helpful at one point in your life may have harmful side effects as you age and your health changes.

Polypharmacy: Too Much of a Good Thing

"Polypharmacy" is a term used to describe the situation where patients, who have multiple medical problems, are prescribed many medications. The more medications an older person takes increases her risk for adverse drug reactions. These reactions can resemble problems that many older people could develop anyway: falling, anxiety, confusion, insomnia, upset stomach, diarrhea, constipation, incontinence, and lack of appetite, among others. Therefore, an adverse drug reaction may go undiagnosed.

This failure to diagnose the drug reaction then causes your loved one to live with yet another distressing symptom that could be relieved by reducing the number of medications she takes. It is not unusual that yet another prescription will be given to combat the new symptoms when actually those symptoms are caused by medication.

For each additional prescription, your loved one takes, there is a 10% increased risk of an adverse reaction. It is easy to see how someone who is prescribed five medications is in great danger of having a complication. If your loved one develops a new symptom, be sure to ask the doctor or APN if the problem could be related to the medications she is taking.

Recommendations for helping a loved one avoid adverse drug reactions include:

- Take an inventory of all medications in the house, and note the date prescribed and expiration dates.

- If possible, ask your loved one if she knows which condition each medication treats and how she takes the medication.

- Make an appointment to see your loved one's primary healthcare provider and bring the list to discuss. At that appointment, verify which prescriptions are current and which medications should be eliminated.

- Ask for an explanation of the benefits and risks of each medication.

- Let the healthcare provider know that it is a goal of yours to avoid adverse drug reactions, and ask if your loved one's medications make her vulnerable to a reaction.

If you are concerned about the prescriptions an older person is taking, a pharmacist is a wonderful resource. Bring the bottles or medication list to the pharmacy and ask to meet with the pharmacist. You can call the pharmacist to request a time to come in for that discussion. Setting up a specific time may ensure that you will have the opportunity to have all your questions answered and not feel rushed. (There are many medications identified as being high-risk medications for older people; see a partial list is in Appendix 5.)

Concerns Regarding Antipsychotic Medications

Antipsychotic medications can cause problems for older people. Although it is common to see antipsychotics used for patients with dementia, it is important to know that this class of drugs remains controversial for these patients. Antipsychotics are approved to treat:

- psychotic disorders
- schizophrenia
- Tourette's syndrome
- bipolar disorders
- other serious neuropsychiatric disorders

Antipsychotic medications for older patients with dementia are considered an "off-label" use of this class of drugs. In other words, it is not a Food and Drug Administration (FDA)-approved practice. Off-label prescribing of drugs is common, though, and can be safe when supported by research that demonstrates a benefit to patients. However, the use of antipsychotic drugs for older people with dementia presents many risks: confusion, anxiety, insomnia, falls resulting in broken hips, heart problems, and increased risk of death. The American Psychiatric Association (APA) has extensive guidelines for prescribing this class of drug to people with dementia. The recommendations include using nondrug interventions to ease the symptoms of dementia before giving antipsychotics.

If there is no improvement in four weeks, after starting antipsychotic drugs, the APA also recommends that the medication slowly be discontinued. Should your loved one be prescribed a new medication to "calm her" or treat her dementia, it is reasonable to speak to the person who prescribed it and discuss those concerns. Be careful to never stop a medication without consulting the prescribing healthcare professional. There can be dramatic complications from suddenly discontinuing some medications—such as severe dizziness, symptoms that can appear to be similar to Parkinson's disease, and dramatic mood disturbances. Always speak with the appropriate doctor or APN before changing medication routines.

Some Common Antipsychotic Medications*

haloperidol (Haldol)	aripiprazole (Abilify)	ziprasidone (Geodon)	lurasidone (Latuda)
olanzapine (Zyprexa)	quetiapine (Seroquel)	risperidone (Risperdal)	clozapine (Clozaril)
asenapine (Saphris)	cariprazine (Vraylar)		

Generic name is followed by the brand name.

Issues with Blood Pressure Medications

If your loved one has been diagnosed with high blood pressure (hypertension) or other cardiovascular diseases, he may be taking a beta-blocker. Beta-blockers are a class of medications that can lower the heart rate and blood pressure and play an important role in preventing complications from hypertension. This type of medication is commonly prescribed for patients who have congestive heart failure.

However, certain beta-blockers have been associated with adding to the likelihood of falls, and that can be related to the dose being taken. These drugs can cause fatigue and dizziness.

When Alma was ninety-five, she grew unusually tired. While that is to be expected at such an advanced age, it still prompted me to take her blood pressure and pulse, although we did not make a habit of checking her vital signs, because her goal was to avoid interventions and doctor's appointments, and monitoring vital signs can lead to a trip on the healthcare conveyor belt. Both her blood pressure and heart rate were extremely low and that could explain her fatigue. I knew that she might be experiencing a side effect of the beta-blocker medication. I called her physician the following day, and over the phone, we agreed that Alma should discontinue taking the beta-blocker. While she still was not running marathons even after removing that medication, she did seem to regain a little more energy.

Some Common Beta-blockers*

labetalol (Normodyne, Trandate)	metoprolol (Lopressor, Toprol)	acebutolol (Sectral) Atenolol	atenolol (Tenormin)
isoprolol (Zebeta)	carvedilol (Coreg)	esmolol (Brevibloc) InnoPran)	propranolol (Inderal)

Generic name is followed by the brand name.

You should never discontinue any medication without speaking to your loved one's physician or other primary healthcare providers. If new symptoms appear, it is worth a discussion with the professionals. It may just require a lower dose to be prescribed for symptoms to improve. If your loved one is of very advanced age, it may even be an opportunity to eliminate one more medication. It is worth a discussion with the doctor or advanced practice nurse.

Vaccinations to Prevent Illness

There are important vaccinations that are recommended for nearly everyone over the age of sixty-five. These vaccines are particularly important for people with multiple medical problems. (See Appendix 3 "Things to Discuss at the Next Medical Appointment" for more specific information.)

Advances in medication can help older people live well, even with multiple medical problems. However, many of these powerful drugs can also lead to additional complications, if not monitored appropriately. It takes active involvement and diligence to be sure your loved one is getting the most from his healthcare. Periodic review of all your loved one's medications is important—even when he is in the care of a skilled nursing or an assisted-living facility. When in doubt, seek professional guidance.

Chapter 11 Key Points

- Multiple medications put your loved one at risk for adverse reactions.

- Review all of her medicines and discuss with her healthcare professional.

- Be aware that there are many medications that need to be used with great caution as people age.

- Question the use of antipsychotics, if your loved one has dementia.

- Ask about what vaccinations are needed.

CHAPTER 12

Maintaining Autonomy: Andy's Story

My brother Andy's story is a lesson in maintaining control over one's healthcare choices. Andy had been living with multiple sclerosis (MS) for more than thirty years by the time I got the call in the middle of the night. At the age of seventy, he lived independently in Nashville and was retired from his professional life.

I had not been aware that Andy was acutely ill until the intensive care doctor called. The doctor needed to know if Andy should be placed on a ventilator. He had been admitted several days earlier with severe anemia and pneumonia and was now not lucid enough to communicate his goals to the staff.

Although Andy and I had not specifically discussed it, I felt he would not want to be on a ventilator. His MS had been progressing, and my experience is that it would be very difficult to get him off a ventilator because of his muscular weakness. Being on a ventilator may have meant he needed sedation and wrist restraints, and those things didn't fit with

Andy's priorities. The ICU doctor asked if antibiotics would be in line with what I knew of Andy's healthcare wishes. I requested that the antibiotics be started. And, I consented to Andy having a BiPAP mask to assist him with his breathing. (BiPAP is similar to the CPAP machines many people wear at night to treat their sleep apnea.) In the meantime, I got on a plane to Nashville.

One Staff Member Can Change Everything

When I arrived, Andy was extremely agitated and trying to remove the BiPAP mask that was helping him breathe. At that moment, a fantastic respiratory therapist (RT) arrived. Her skill and compassion were both truly amazing. Rather than taking the usual "You have to leave the mask on" approach, she offered to take the mask off. She replaced the mask with a high flow nasal cannula. Although it would not assist his breathing effort, it would deliver much-needed oxygen to him.

When the respiratory therapist took off the mask, Andy stated clearly, "And leave it off!" Andy relaxed as soon as the mask was off. There was no more agitation, and he was able to rest.

This incident raises an important issue. The way a single staff member handles a situation can set the course for a patient's hospitalization. Had a different respiratory therapist come into his room that night and seen Andy removing the BiPAP mask, that RT may have called the nurse, who would then have gotten an order to put restraints on Andy to prevent him from removing the mask. He very well could have either had restraints put on his wrists or been prescribed sedation to keep him from being agitated. These sorts of decisions are made every day in hospitals. They are not done with the intent to harm or frighten patients; on the contrary, they are done to help facilitate the treatments that have been determined necessary. However, interventions done with the best of intentions can also be harmful. These situations might cause an escalation of interventions and treatments that may not have been necessary if the staff looked at things from the patient's perspective. This, again, illustrates the importance of having clear goals and someone who can advocate for those goals. Frequently, ICU doctors and nurses are conflicted by starting ever-increasingly aggressive treatments, but, without clear direction from the patient or his family, they feel obligated to continue.

Two days later, Andy was a new man. The antibiotics had controlled his pneumonia, and he was awake and alert. Pneumonia had started from an aspiration problem. Andy's swallow was not strong enough to keep small amounts of liquid and food from going into his lungs. That led to aspiration pneumonia, and the bacterial infection started from his weakened immunity. The fluid that had accumulated in his lungs was the medium for the infection. This led the doctors to suggest that Andy undergo a procedure to insert a feeding tube through his abdomen into his stomach. After that, he would have liquid feedings (tube-feeding) that would be given through the tube.

Feeding Tubes and Personal Choices

Many people have a feeding tube. Often, patients get them after a stroke has made swallowing food difficult; it is a common and simple procedure. But, Andy declined the tube-feeding recommendation because so much of his life was already restricted. He could no longer walk or even use his hands for detailed tasks—needing help to put on a shirt, for instance. He knew that eating and drinking were two physical pleasures he still controlled, and he was not willing to lose them. This, of course, made the doctors frown; they are used to having their suggestions followed. But, Andy is extremely competent and was determined to keep control of his treatment. He understood the risks and was willing to face the consequences of another pneumonia rather than to have a feeding tube.

If your loved one is frail and has multiple medical problems but can still find enjoyment in a candy bar or ice cream soda or perhaps even a glass of wine or order of French fries, I encourage you to give careful thought before consenting to a feeding tube.

This is a common scenario: An elderly patient with dementia is brought to the hospital with a report of mental status changes, and she has stopped eating and drinking. After the initial crisis is managed, it is discovered that her swallow is weak; maybe she is coughing after a sip of water, for example. Speech pathologists come in to do a swallow study to evaluate it. If in their professional judgment, her swallow is putting her at risk for aspiration, they will make recommendations. Sometimes the advice is to allow the patient to have only thick fluids (People are more likely to choke and cough when swallowing water, rather than a smoothie.). If this is the case, then powder thickeners are added to any thin liquids until the patient's swallow is stronger.

But, many times, it is determined that it is unlikely the patient will regain a stronger swallow, and a feeding tube is recommended. It is a minor procedure; a soft tube is inserted through a small incision in the abdomen into the stomach or just past the stomach into the small intestine. A local anesthetic is used, and intravenous sedation is given for the procedure. This feeding-tube insertion is frequently one stop on the healthcare conveyor belt for some patients.

Too often, the patient's quality of life after the tube is put in is not considered. Of course, if the patient is capable of making her own decision, she should decide. But, often it is a family member who must approve the surgery. And, if we phrase it as, "Your grandmother will choke on her food and likely get pneumonia, which may kill her," then, of course, family members will consent to the feeding tube. This can be an example of "misinformed consent."

Instead, if we encourage family members to think about whether the pleasures of eating and drinking are important at this stage of life, perhaps different decisions would be made. If you are unable to walk independently, unable to manage most of your affairs or living situation, and perhaps unable to enjoy reading or watching television due to a decreasing memory and attention span, would eating and drinking take on an added importance as a remaining pleasure in your life? It is something to consider.

However, there are patients who will not be able to enjoy eating or drinking. Some of these are patients who have stopped eating because they have advanced stage dementia, end-stage cancer, or other medical conditions. Feeding tubes are a complex issue when caring for these patients.

Again, I encourage you to determine the goal for this procedure. What is there to be gained in putting in a feeding tube? Like every intervention we do, feeding tubes can lead to negative consequences, including infection, aspiration of the tube feeding into the lungs, and chronic diarrhea. As we saw in Chapter 7, feeding tubes also make it more likely that someone with dementia will have her hands and wrists restrained to keep her from pulling on the tube. Restraining someone in this way can have many unwanted effects.

It is important to remember that feeding tubes can be an appropriate option for some patients. They allow a patient, who has an inability to swallow, to take medications and get the nutrition that otherwise would not be possible. My point here is not that feeding tubes are always bad, but that we need to have our goals understood, and that will make these decisions easier for our own and our loved ones' healthcare. It is also essential to remember that, when faced with the prospect of any intervention, it is wise to ask:

- **What complications can happen?** Nausea is common with feeding tubes; bleeding and infection can occur. When you ask about complications, be sure that you are asking about the complications *during* surgery as well as those that are likely *after* surgery. You will want to ask about the complications for people who are living with a feeding tube.

- **What are the long-term complications that someone with her medical history is vulnerable to?** It is important to ask the healthcare professionals to consider your loved one's specific risks for any treatment or intervention.

Staying in Charge and Choosing
Heart Valve Surgery

It has been a few years since that middle-of-the-night call, and Andy is doing as well as can be expected for someone with advanced MS. During that hospitalization, he was diagnosed with a heart-valve problem that can cause sudden death. It is possible to get a valve replacement, and now, several years after he had been critically ill, Andy considered the risks and benefits of having that surgery.

Many people in his situation (or people trying to put themselves in his place) would say "no" to the surgery. Given his fragile condition, any surgery has a risk for complications. But, Andy was hoping that the heart-valve surgery might improve his energy levels. He knew the risks and had done a lot of reading about his heart-valve diagnosis.

Andy had the surgery, and it was uncomplicated, although he has not noticed the hoped-for increase in stamina. He is still very much in charge of his life and clear about his goals. In spite of that, I am sure that new staff at the facility who see this white-haired, frail man in his seventies with advanced multiple sclerosis in a wheelchair, view him differently. Their expectations may be that he will be passive or depressed.

Wrong Assumptions Can Lead to Misdiagnosis

Andy remains one of the most intelligent, quick-minded people I have ever known. His intellect has not been affected by MS. Because of this, he is not necessarily interested in the typical activities that are scheduled in most skilled-care facilities. He describes them as: "A group of people sitting in chairs and staring at someone talking at the front of the room."

That has been my experience when I visit. Even though he is in what is described as a "five-star" facility, the social events are primarily bingo or activities more often seen in a kindergarten class. Singing songs or doing craft projects is common. While there is nothing wrong with these events, they are not particularly interesting to a man who is intellectually active, even while his body is failing him. He would love to have discussions with other residents about current affairs, for example, but instead of news programs, the televisions are usually on game shows. Many of the residents do not have the attention span necessary for more-involved or complex programs.

Apparently, the social worker became concerned that Andy was not participating in what she considered appropriate social activities. Mentally, Andy is more on the level of the residents in the independent or assisted-living parts of the building. Unfortunately, the policy is to keep the skilled nursing residents completely separate from the other residents; therefore, he cannot get that social interaction.

The social worker made a referral requesting that the staff psychiatrist see Andy. In an absurd turn of events, the psychiatrist wrote a report stating that Andy was "inappropriately optimistic about his condition." Having expected to meet with a depressed patient, apparently, the psychiatrist was unable to see past his expectations when he found an alert and engaged conversationalist. Instead of suggesting that Andy have more appropriate activity options, the doctor found a pathology in Andy's optimism.

The doctor also stated that the staff reported Andy could be grumpy or confrontational. This probably, in part, results from his insistence the staff tells him what medication they are giving him and what conditions they are treating. Often, we, in the healthcare field, encourage people to be involved in their own care, to ask questions and take ownership of their health. But, I have found that patients who are viewed as weak, frail and dependent are expected to be passive in their interactions with doctors, nurses and nursing assistants.

More than once, Andy has experienced the staff trying to administer the incorrect medication or the wrong dose of medication to him. Human beings make mistakes, which is why it is important for patients to ask questions. But it seems the staff inaccurately interpreted Andy's questions as hostile or inappropriate. That impression was passed on to the psychiatrist, who did not consider Andy's entire situation or individual circumstances. This is an example of "the system" refusing to see things from the patient's perspective.

Andy's story highlights the need for people to have a clear idea of their individual goals for healthcare. Without those goals, it is very easy to be swept up into the healthcare conveyor belt system and have your choices taken away. Having a clear sense of his goals helped Andy to maintain his autonomy, even in the presence of a profound disability.

Chapter 12 Key Points

- Remember that you or your loved one are free to question any treatments or medical orders. If Andy had been less assertive, he would have kept that BiPAP mask on. He also would have gotten a feeding tube that would have deprived him of the simple pleasure of eating for several years, as well as exposed him to complications from the tube.

- No one single surgery, procedure or medication is right for everyone. In Andy's particular circumstances, the feeding tube was rejected, but heart-valve surgery was accepted. This is what fits in with his goals and values.

- Supporting your loved one in his medical decisions is important. Having the heart-valve surgery posed significant risks; knowing the risks, Andy decided to proceed with it. It was my job to support him in that decision.

- Help the healthcare providers see your loved one as an individual with unique needs and values, rather than a list of medical diagnoses. Have conversations with the medical staff, and let them know personal details of your loved one's life; bring in family photos and help the staff see the human being instead of the illness.

Helping the staff to see your loved one in this way may prevent incorrect assumptions or a misdiagnosis when he doesn't follow an expected pattern of behavior.

CHAPTER 13

When a Younger Patient Revises His Goals: Mike's Story

A year or so after my mother died, my ex-husband became gravely ill. I had known that Mike was not feeling well. We divorced twenty years ago, and, although we both continued to live near one another on the South Side of Chicago, I had not seen him for several months. Still, we had kept in touch, and he had recently been texting me about some health issues.

Trained as a lawyer, Mike had been an associate professor of criminal law and public safety at a small college for the past fifteen years. He loved his work, and I was concerned to hear that he had not been teaching for a few months after having had a minor surgical procedure. He was plagued with constant pains in his legs, and I was encouraging him to see his doctor as soon as possible.

One autumn morning, our daughter called from her home in Los Angeles. I had barely said hello when Katie's distressed voice said, "Dad's in the hospital." Katie had gotten word that Mike was in the ER of a hospital near the college where he taught. I tried to reassure her that I had talked to her dad the night before and had told him to see a doctor as soon as possible. I assumed he was following that advice. But, I knew that Katie needed me to go to the hospital to be sure that he was well taken care of. And so, began a heartbreaking eight-week journey.

The Initial Goal

It was a thirty-minute drive to the hospital. On my way, I called Mike's personal physician whom I had known for several years. I wanted to let her know that Mike was in the ER of a small community hospital, and I was asking for her help. If he needed to be hospitalized, I asked her to transfer him to the large teaching hospital where she had admitting privileges. She assured me she would and said she would call the ER to inquire about his status.

Mike always listed her as his primary physician, so I did not worry about confidentiality rules preventing an exchange of information. She called me back as I was walking into the ER where Mike was being seen and told me the devastating results of his blood tests. His hemoglobin was dangerously low, and he would be prone to catastrophic bleeding due to his blood not clotting properly. Dr. Hagan went on to say, "Margaret, Mike will not be able to be transferred anytime soon." I thanked her and said I would be in touch with her. Doctors like her are few and far between. Dr. Vanessa Hagan had been a valuable person for Mike and for my mother years earlier. I was grateful to know her.

Even that conversation with Dr. Hagan did not prepare me for what I saw when I entered the ER that morning. Mike has always been a friendly, outgoing person, so I expected to hear him joking with a doctor or engaged in a political debate with a nurse. Instead, he was barely responsive and extremely jaundiced. My experience in caring for patients waiting for liver transplants made me fear that Mike was in liver failure. I walked over to him, brushed the hair from his eyes, and told him I was there. He started to move his hands as if he wanted to write something, even though he could not open his eyes. I handed him a pen and held paper for him, but he was too confused and weak even to hold the pen, let alone to write. I told him to rest and that we would take care of everything.

At this point, what was the goal? To save the life of this dynamic fifty-four-year-old man, who had so much to live for, and whom I assumed had many more years to live. Within a few minutes of my arrival, the doctors showed me Mike's blood tests, which confirmed the liver failure. Because Mike was barely responsive, and we knew from the lab results that his condition was likely to worsen before it could get better; so, we agreed he needed a breathing tube and to be on a ventilator.

Within a few hours, Mike was in the ICU in critical condition, and Katie, along with our son, Peter, were both flying in from Los Angeles. Mike had a gregarious personality and many friends, none better than Michele and Dan, who worked with him for many years at the college. They were with me in the ER that day and nearly every day for the eight weeks that Mike struggled for his life. They helped with updating concerned coworkers at the college, as well as navigating some insurance issues that came up.

Our goal was clear: Get Mike past this immediate threat and learn how to get him on the road to good health. That is what drove every decision for the next few weeks, even though my conversations with the critical-care physician were not encouraging. After a week in the ICU, Mike was still not fully awake. In response to our question regarding Mike's prognosis, the critical-care specialist said, "Well, if you want to talk about rainbows and unicorns, I would say we need to get him out of this acute phase of the illness for at least six months and put him on the liver transplant list. If you want me to be realistic, it is unlikely he will live that long."

The words Mike's critical-care doctor used may seem unnecessarily harsh, but I appreciated his candor. I know from my professional experience, that even when we are very blunt about a patient's dire circumstances, family members are often overly optimistic. The reality can be too painful. It can take many conversations over several days for family members to fully grasp the severity of a patient's illness. It is so difficult for people to realize that, even with all of our advanced knowledge and technology, there are limits to what we can do to restore a patient to health.

Having Power of Attorney

For most of the next seven weeks, Mike was in the ICU, but he had regained consciousness and was able to communicate with us. Having been a nurse in an ICU of a liver-transplant program years earlier, I knew how devastating liver disease could be, and that drove me to encourage Mike to get his affairs in order.

What is it they say about the cobbler's children going barefoot? Well, Mike was an attorney without a Will or Trust. After about ten days, he was able to speak with a lawyer who was kind enough to come to the hospital. During that visit, Mike dictated the terms of his will and trust. We also signed the power of attorney papers for both healthcare and financial matters. It allowed me access to his bank accounts and officially made me his healthcare power of attorney.

I have to confess that, up until that point, I had no actual paperwork stating I was the decision-maker. It is a technical issue because as next of kin, Peter and Katie would have been looked to for the decisions when Mike was unable to communicate. But that devastating day in the ER, I told the doctors that I was Mike's healthcare power of attorney. Although we were divorced, Mike had always looked to me for help with medical issues, just as I had used his legal expertise when I needed it. I knew that Peter and Katie were not in an emotional state to be making decisions for their father, and I trusted that I knew him well enough to assume he would want me to step in. The kids agreed.

As it turns out, Mike told me later that when he was motioning for a pen to write in the ER that first day, he had wanted to write a note. "Margaret, I was trying to tell them to listen to you." I was thankful that he trusted me in that way. But, do not put yourself in that position. Do everything you can to have those loved ones closest to you complete necessary paperwork establishing who the decision-maker will be if they are critically ill or injured.

Once I had the official paperwork, the kids and I could start the process of making renovations to Mike's home in preparation for him to return. As a bachelor for the past twenty years, he had not updated his home in ways that would have made it easy for him to recuperate there from a long illness, so we set out to make that happen. But in the ensuing weeks, with so many setbacks and no real improvement, it became apparent that Mike would not be returning to that home.

Prepare for the Worst and Hope for the Best

We were fortunate that Mike re-gained consciousness. Without the will and trust and the official POA documents, the following weeks and months would have been more complicated. Get the legal matters settled early on in the process of a serious illness. It can seem like the last thing you want to deal with when you are focused on a loved one whose life is in the balance. But, if you do not secure access to bank accounts and the proper powers of attorney, you will have much more stress.

This is an area where you can accept the offers of help from close friends or family. This is when you need to ask a trusted person to gather information about what has to be done and to contact a lawyer to help if needed. (See Appendix 2 for a list of important documents to gather.)

For a younger person, a sudden illness can catch everyone off-guard. Even being a lawyer, Mike did not have his legal affairs in order. Do not assume that these issues are taken care of, no matter how close you are to the person. Your loved ones with chronic illnesses should be encouraged to complete powers of attorney for financial affairs, as well as for healthcare. This should be done *before* a health crisis occurs. Doing these things is an act of love and caring that they can do for you because you will be the one who suffers if these vital issues are not resolved.

Even for those of us for whom chronic illness seems an unlikely scenario, a tragic accident can happen at any time. In the U.S. in 2015, for example, more than 1 million people between the ages of thirty and sixty were injured in car accidents alone. Surely, most of the million people had no idea at the start of the day that they would be in the ER by day's end. More than 16,000 of those people died as a result of their injuries. This illustrates how vital it is to prepare for a situation wherein you are incapacitated for even a brief period of time. Having the proper preparation, such as POAs and electronic bill pay, as well as a Will and Trust, will help make the trauma less devastating for those you love.

If you are helping someone who has a sudden serious illness, try to set up automatic payments for their important bills, such as rent/mortgage, utilities, insurance, and any other bill that would cause problems if the payments were not made. While there will not be devastating consequences if the cable bill does not get paid, if insurance is interrupted or foreclosure for nonpayment of mortgage occurs, you will have another crisis on your hands.

Several weeks passed without substantial improvement, and the doctors suggested that Mike be transferred to a major university medical center in Chicago. Although we had grown to love and trust the staff at the community hospital, we all felt the resources at a larger institution would be of benefit. Unfortunately, even with all the brilliant, highly trained, and acclaimed staff, Mike was still not improving. He was suffering from frequent episodes of internal bleeding. There was never a three-day period in which he did not require a blood transfusion just to keep his blood count in an acceptably low range.

After several more weeks of suffering and no improvement, the doctors gave us a choice to continue on the present course or seek hospice care, which is directed toward comfort rather than cure.

Choosing Hospice: A New Goal

Peter, Katie and I did not want to make the decision about changing to hospice. Mike had many days where he was too sleepy to talk and could not interact with us. We asked the doctors to schedule a meeting where the team could come in and speak with us. Peter and Katie flew in from LA, and we were fortunate that Mike had a rare day of being alert and awake the day of the meeting, and he was the central participant. This meeting became another opportunity for us to clarify the goals for Mike's care.

After listening to the doctors, Mike turned to each of us for our opinions. I have to admit I feel I let him down that day. Sitting there, holding Peter and Katie's hands, when Mike asked what I thought of him choosing hospice care over continuing the current aggressive treatment, I broke down in tears. The regret I have about how I handled that day will never leave me. Although, I know that Mike made a choice he needed to make. It was the choice that acknowledged the reality that the rainbows and unicorns were never going to come. But I wish I was better able to help him make that choice. I wish that I had asked the doctors this critical question: "If Mike were *your* fifty-four-year-old father or uncle or brother, someone you loved, what is the advice you would give to him?"

I am confident that they would have recommended hospice care over continuing the likely futile cycle of blood transfusions and pain. They knew that maintaining the current course was becoming increasingly ineffective, and Mike was likely to have a bleeding episode that could cause cardiac arrest, meaning a "code" would be called, resulting in CPR, and being put on a ventilator with little hope of recovery. Still, I regret having gone into that day ill-prepared for my emotions.

Mike had not been allowed to eat or drink (called an NPO order) for two days because he was too weak to swallow effectively. He needed more blood transfusions and was possibly going to have another procedure to try to stop the internal bleeding. He was in constant pain because giving him narcotics caused his blood pressure to drop to dangerously low levels. All of that suffering could be alleviated with hospice care.

Hospice care has the goal of providing comfort and improving the quality of life for the patient and the family, rather than curing the illness. His first question about changing to hospice care was, "Does that mean I can drink water?" He was reassured to hear that he could and relieved to know that pain medication would not be withheld based on his vital signs. At that point, Mike turned to us and clearly said, "Then I want hospice."

Mike was transferred to an in-patient hospice unit because he was too weak to be at home. One goal now was that he would get to go home, but we all knew that was unlikely. The primary goal became his comfort. Within forty-eight hours of being in hospice, Mike died. He was peaceful and knew that we were all there with him. This was a heartbreaking loss for all of us, but especially for Peter and Katie, who lost their dad much too soon.

Even with all my experience in working with critically ill patients, there were things I neglected to do for Mike. In hindsight, I realize how the stress of the situation gave me tunnel vision, and I simply could not see the big picture. If I could do it over, I would have asked for a palliative-care specialist to evaluate Mike early on in his struggle. Palliative care could have been added to the aggressive treatments and certainly would have helped Mike be more comfortable over those weeks. Thinking back on this, it is unimaginable that I did not think of this—and that no one offered it.

This is a stark example of how we get tunnel vision in these circumstances. If you think you are too close to the situation, ask a friend or a trusted person, who is not entangled with all the personal issues, to help you to look at the overall picture. A fresh perspective from another person may give you ideas that your exhaustion kept you from seeing.

Ho'oponopono: I Love You, I'm Sorry, Please Forgive Me

Still, we are grateful for the time we all had together in those trying weeks. Knowing that people lose loved ones suddenly without having had the chance to spend many hours together, I am grateful that, if we had to lose Mike, at least we had the opportunity to share moments at the end of his life. One of the precious moments came a day before he made the decision to go into hospice care. I cannot remember where I had heard about the South Pacific Island tradition of Ho'oponopono, which includes practices of forgiveness and reconciliation, but I thought it might help bring Mike peace. It encourages people to say, "I love you. I'm sorry. Please forgive me. Thank you."

I sat with him and asked him to tell Peter and Katie how much he loved them and that he was sorry for not always being the father they deserved. I expected that he would agree but thought he would have that conversation with them when they came back into town. Instead, he looked at me and said, "Yes, let's get them on the phone right now." His immediate response shocked me, but I realize now that he knew that his life was coming to an end.

Up to that point, we had not talked of pursuing hospice care; when he was awake enough, he often spoke of planning his recovery. But, he wanted to take advantage of this moment, and so we called the kids. Mike told them how much he loved them, that he was proud to be their father, and he hoped they could forgive him for letting them down.

When I suggested that Mike have that talk with our kids, I was hesitant because I was unsure how he would react. Now, I am so grateful that I took the chance. It gave him a precious opportunity to have important conversations with Peter and Katie. It would have been tragic if they missed out on that experience. If you find yourself in a similar situation, try to find time for healing. Most of us have issues that need healing with even the most cherished loved one. Making it an intentional conversation will be a gift for both of you.

Although Mike did not have a long time to get the benefits of hospice care, he was in control of the choices. He made the decision to stop pursuing what appeared to be a futile goal of recovery and to have a death that was peaceful, rather than in the frenetic atmosphere of the ICU.

Taking Care of Yourself as the Caregiver

If Mike had made a different choice the next day when speaking to the doctors, if he had said he still wanted aggressive treatment in the hope of recovery, I would have supported him. It would have been difficult, though, because the weeks of bedside vigil and the responsibilities I carried were exhausting. It was becoming clear that all of his suffering was not going to lead to his recovery. This situation was taking its toll.

My husband, Jim, is an exceptionally patient person, but even he was pushed to the limit by my spending most of my days off work at either the hospital or Mike's house taking care of things there. There is no shortage of advice for people taking care of a loved one: *Care for yourself, take time away, etc.* But, when you are in the midst of the storm, it is hard to step back and also difficult to take oneself off high alert and relax. I will always be grateful to Jim for his support and patience.

I know we could not have gotten through this difficult journey with Mike without the support of Michele and Dan, his devoted friends. That kind of emotional and practical support is essential when going through this sort of situation.

Mike's brother and sister, along with their mother, Judy, were a constant source of love, even in their own deep grief.

Take the life preservers that are thrown your way when you are drifting out to sea. You will have the chance to do the same for someone else at another time in your life. Here are some ideas for ways people can help:

- Ask someone to make phone calls for you, if you need information about extended care or other details that do not require your immediate attention. These sort of telephone or Internet-based research tasks can even be done by someone who is living in another state but who wants to help.

- Do you have dry cleaning or groceries that need to be picked up? Ask someone to do it for you.

- Do you have children that need chauffeuring? Or, is there another family member that needs visiting or other attention during the crisis? Does your grass need cutting or snow need shoveling? If a neighbor or friend offers to help you, they can easily do this for you.

Reach out for and accept all of the love and support that you can during these times. Without it, you may very well become the next patient.

Chapter 13 Key Points

- **Palliative Care:** Ask about it as soon as possible. If the hospital does not have a specific palliative-care department, ask if you can speak to someone who directs hospice care. You may not want specific "end of life" care offered by hospice, but the physicians and nurses who work in hospice are experts at symptom control. They can help with suggestions for how your loved one can be more comfortable while aggressive treatments are given.

- **Ho'oponopono:** If you or a loved one becomes suddenly ill, consider this practice, which can bring healing to family and friends.

- **Powers of Attorney, Banking and Paying the Bills:** Sudden death, severe illness or injury can happen to anyone at any time. Do your family and loved ones a kindness and have your financial and legal planning in order. See Appendix 2 for a specific list of suggestions.

- **Self-Care:** If you find yourself in a similar circum-stance, accept the help offered. It takes a willingness to be vulnerable to welcome a helping hand, rather than trying to "suck it up" and go it alone.

CHAPTER 14

Lessons Learned

If you are caring for an aging loved one, this may be one of the most stressful, yet rewarding, times in your life. I have spoken to many people caring for their parents, another relative, or friend, and a common theme comes up: This is a precious time in which to deepen the relationship. It can be a unique time when you come to know this relative on a completely different level than you had before. And yet, it is also undeniably stressful. Being responsible for another adult's care has many challenges. It is a time that can drain your financial and emotional resources, as well as impact your own health.

The Perils of Parenting Your Parent

I have referenced many resources in this book, and I encourage you to use them. There are services that can be of assistance, but it does take persistence to access them. There are also things that you can keep in mind to lower your stress and that of your loved one. Try to remember that you are dealing with an adult.

It is tempting to think of caring for an aging parent as switching roles. It is especially true when there is an element of dementia, and you find yourself being responsible for not just financial affairs, but also the physical care of your parent. I would encourage you to resist the inclination to view your parent as a child. Having the point of view that you are now "parenting your parent" can set you up for conflicts. Having a parental approach to your aging loved one robs her of the place she has earned in the world. It can also set up disagreements to be a test of wills, rather than an opportunity for compromise.

Everyone's situation in caregiving is unique. I realize that some people who are trying to care for parents with profound dementia must deal with behavioral disorders, anger, and sometimes even violence. These are difficult circumstances, and if your approach is working for you and your loved one, then stay your course. But, if it is not working, if you find yourself arguing and stressed, I encourage you to implement another strategy.

Frequently, when people lash out in anger, they are in their self-protection mode. What seems like an unreasonable burst of anger may be caused by your loved one feeling out of control or threatened in some way. Needing the help of another person for even the most basic tasks in life puts anyone in a vulnerable place. It is likely that most choices have been taken away, either by physical limitations or other practical reasons. This lack of control can cause her to lash out. Because you are the one closest, you are the likely target. If there is a way that you can provide your loved one with choices while trying to keep her personal preferences in mind, you may have success in preventing an upset.

Even with the best advice and support, caring for an aging loved one is a challenging experience. My sister said it best: "Daughter guilt is worse than parent guilt." By that, she meant to say that as much as we feel we could do things better for our children and stress over our mistakes, the reality of being responsible for our mother carried more guilt and anxiety. But, with planning and open communication, it is possible to feel that you have done the best you could and be content with the outcome.

Give the Gift of Asking About Goals and Values

Each situation is different, and each carries its own struggles. In my experience, both personally and professionally, planning and communication hold the keys to a lower stress level.

Using the suggestions and resources in this book will help you clarify your goals and values surrounding healthcare decisions.

We Can Do Better for the Most Vulnerable Among Us

I carry with me the image of Mr. Johnson, who had died in the ICU after going through the code process and being on a ventilator. At eighty years old and with advanced lung cancer, Mr. Johnson died with wrist restraints on his arms, so he would not pull on his breathing tube. He died in an unfamiliar place that was ill-equipped to help him and his family deal with one of the most significant times in their lives. Mr. Johnson and his entire family needlessly suffered because they were on the healthcare conveyor belt.

We can do better than this for the most vulnerable among us, but it will happen only when each of us advocates for the people we love. That advocacy starts with understanding our loved one's goals and values. It starts with asking and listening—something each of us can do for one another. The suffering that will be prevented will be well worth the effort.

When speaking to your loved ones or other family members about setting their healthcare goals, you can shape it as a request for help. Ask for your loved one to help you understand how to represent his goals and values. You cannot understand them if you do not know what they are. Even if you have a vague idea from family conversations or an understanding of your loved one's religious beliefs, goals and values evolve over the years. With advancing age and when new medical issues arise, perspectives change, and your loved one may have a different outlook on healthcare issues now. Give him the opportunity to share his thoughts with you.

Alma: A Beautiful Life

In the weeks after her ninety-ninth birthday, Alma started to feel weaker. Although she laughed every day and was a pleasure to be with, she was clearly not feeling well. As we prepared weeks earlier for her birthday party, more than once she said that it would be her last birthday. She didn't say it with sadness or regret; it was more matter-of-fact. She was tired and felt it was time for her life to conclude. I regret that I did not explore those feelings with her more. The thought that she wouldn't be with us was not something I wanted to accept as a reality. I am a healthcare professional, and I have been at the bedsides of many people as they approached the end of their lives. Yet, this, of course, was different. This was my mother.

In the last three days of her life, she slept more and stayed in bed. I suspected that she had pneumonia, but I knew she did not want antibiotics. They always gave her nausea, and that was something she did not want to feel at this point. And I knew that she wanted to be at home. And so, Peter and Katie were able to spend time with her in a peaceful setting, as was I, in those final two days. My sister, Rita, came, and Mother sat up in bed and said: "Oh, Rita, I'm not feeling well." She knew Rita was there, and it was a comfort to her.

While I knew I would experience great grief in the loss of my mother, I was comforted by knowing that I had honored her wishes for those last few years. Even at ninety-nine years old, her autonomy and dignity were respected because we knew her goals and values.

Throughout that last evening, I was on the phone and also texting various family members. I knew that we were probably in the final days of her life. It seemed surreal to imagine our large extended family—now including 23 grandchildren and 13 great-grandchildren—without Alma to lead us.

I think now of how my niece, with tears in her eyes, recently told me how sad she is that "Grandma Alma would never hold Hayes," my new great-nephew. It is hard to imagine her not having the chance to hold this precious baby. We all took joy in watching Mother's love and enthusiasm for each new baby. She provided so much guidance overtly as well as by example and we can only hope to carry on her legacy.

Later that evening, Mother woke and asked me to help her to turn on her side. Rearranging her pillows, I made sure she had her rosary and handkerchief. Those were two things that she always had with her in bed. I left Mother's room to set up coffee for the morning since I knew my brothers and sisters would be coming early to be with her. When I returned to her room, I realized that she had died. She was peaceful and comfortable in the end, in familiar surroundings, and as she had planned. A beautiful life from beginning to end.

Chapter 14 Key Points

- Acknowledging and planning for the fact that all of our lives will come to an end is not morbid and need not be sad. Making plans and having the conversation with the relevant people is an act of love we can share.

- Remember that you are trying to understand how your loved one wants to live the last part of her life. This is as much about living and staying off the healthcare conveyor belt as it is about preparing for the end of life.

- A summary of all the chapters' Key Points can be found in Appendix 6.

Appendix 1

To Go or Not To Go To the ER: A Decision Guide

This is a question that can cause great stress when caring for a loved one. New symptoms come up, and it always seems to be after 5:00 p.m. on a Friday when they do. I have created a flowchart guide that can help you when you are in the situation not knowing whether to call 911 or wait until you can reach your healthcare provider.

The flowchart guide could not be printed in this book due to sizing and formatting issues. However, it is currently available online. If you go to *GettingTheBestCare.com*, you will be able to get a free copy of this vital guide. This will help you so that each new symptom does not cause a crisis.

Appendix 2

Why a Power of Attorney May Not Have Power

This book is primarily about how to navigate all the choices you will face—for healthcare—while helping an aging loved one. But, unfortunately, a personal tragedy prompts me to add something regarding legal planning as we age.

One of my dear friends recently had a cardiac arrest in his home at the age of seventy-five and was resuscitated by paramedics. As the statistics showed us earlier in the book, the chance of Phil making a meaningful recovery after having an out-of-hospital cardiac arrest was very low. As it turned out, after four days of intensive care, the tests showed that he had suffered a devastating brain injury that was not survivable. We made the decision to withdraw the ventilator and allow Phil to die peacefully.

What we could not control, however, was the legal and financial planning that he had done years earlier. I am grateful that Phil gave me co-power of attorney for healthcare, along with his son. But, he clearly did not have the best or most up-to-date advice regarding financial planning.

Because he had been very successful, Phil was able to retire early and still had considerable wealth when he died. He had lived a frugal life and had invested well. Unfortunately, the only instructions left regarding his wealth were included in a Will. It is easy to assume that a Will is sufficient to help your surviving loved ones to manage your finances and property after you die. However, this experience has demonstrated that it is not enough.

If you have only a Will, it requires all of your assets to be put into probate after you die. The details of what that means can be learned elsewhere. Suffice it to say, having all of your assets in probate court for many months prevents your loved ones from using even your checking account to pay bills or to provide for the immediate needs of your children or other dependents. This can create great stress and frustration for those you love.

A more useful document to have is a Trust. When you establish a Trust, there is no need to have a court to oversee those assets after you die. The people you name in the Trust are able to act on your stated wishes immediately to care for your dependents and manage other financial obligations, such as your burial or other final arrangements.

I cannot pretend to understand all of the details of having a Will and Trust. But, I wanted to give you this warning because, after it was determined that Phil could not survive, the primary stress I experienced was regarding how to provide for the needs of his dependents. I knew that there was nothing medically to be done, and I could make peace with that fact. But, the ill-planned financial situation created an enormous strain on us emotionally. Please, do all you can to secure your assets after you die and to make things as stress-free as possible for those you love. None of us knows when we will die.

My friend certainly did not plan to have a sudden cardiac arrest on that Sunday morning, but such a crisis could happen to anyone. We would all be wise to stop now and be sure to establish:

- **Healthcare power of attorney,** so that there is a designated person to make the decisions with your physicians. Some people advise that you have two friends or family members be "co-powers" of attorney for healthcare. They reason that having two people is a good idea so that they will help one another shoulder the stress of important decisions. I disagree with this strategy. It sounds good, in theory, but problems can arise. It requires both to be present when needed and in agreement. You cannot predict how the stress of the situation will affect others, and two people who usually are of the same opinion can suddenly have very different views on life and death decisions. This can create a stalemate that can set them up for an emotional upset, as well as leave the healthcare providers guessing as to who is making the final decisions. I think a better way is to appoint successive powers of attorney for healthcare, as well as for finances. For example, if you list your spouse as POA, but your spouse is unable or unwilling to perform the duties, he can decline, and a successor POA will step in. If the successor is unavailable or unable/unwilling to be the POA, the third successor steps in. This way, you have a contingency plan, if your original POA choice cannot carry out the duties. You have a plan in place that allows for changing circumstances.

- **Financial power of attorney,** so that if you are incapacitated, bills can be paid and your financial affairs tended to until you are able to do so.

- **Will and Trust,** so that your loved ones will not have to endure the delays and the expenses that go with having all of your assets in probate court.

Even if you are a person with modest means, having a Will and Trust is necessary in order for your loved ones to be able to manage even a small checking or savings account, mortgage payments, electric bills, and a funeral. A financial power of attorney does not have any legal standing after the person dies. Do not think that because you have a financial POA established that will allow your loved ones to make financial decisions after you die. A power of attorney expires when you die.

A Caution Regarding Financial Power of Attorney

My friend, Phil probably felt that he had diligently completed the necessary paperwork when he put together his Will and the healthcare and financial powers of attorney. Unfortunately, The financial power of attorney proved insufficient to give us immediate access to his checking account.

Even though the power of attorney was legal and proper for the state of California where he lived, his bank required more. We learned that financial institutions (such as banks, credit unions, and investment firms) frequently would not honor the power of attorney, alone. They require that you have forms specific to their institution, in addition to the POA. It had been too late for us because Phil was already incapacitated when we learned we needed the bank forms. Essentially, the POA form was useless to help us when we needed immediate access to cash.

You Need These Things:

- Healthcare power of attorney
- Advance directive, which makes your goals and values for healthcare clear (see Prepareforyourcare.org and TheConversationProject.org)
- Financial power of attorney bank-specific forms for POA
- Social Security forms for POA
- Veterans Administration forms for POA (if applicable)
- Investment house form for POA (if applicable)

What is needed to prevent added expense and delays after you die:

- Will and Trust
- A written statement telling your loved ones your preferences for and any arrangements you have made for burial or cremation.

Take time to clarify your goals and values regarding healthcare. Additionally, do all those you love a kindness by having a POA for healthcare and for financial matters, and also you need to consider a Will and a Trust. Losing a cherished family member or friend is extremely stressful. Do all you can to help the people you love to avoid additional stress by preparing now.

Appendix 3

Things to Discuss at the Next Medical Appointment

Here are some things to keep in mind the next time you accompany your loved one to see her doctor or advance practice nurse.

Goals

Be prepared to discuss your loved one's goals for healthcare. If avoiding doctor's appointments, blood testing, and other interventions is important to your loved one, be sure to let your healthcare provider know, and ask for help in achieving the goals. For instance, there are certain symptoms to watch for if your loved one has heart failure, diabetes or kidney failure. If the symptoms are noticed at an early stage, effective treatment can happen at home and prevent a disruptive trip to the emergency room. Take the opportunity to ask your healthcare provider for tips about what to watch for, regarding your loved one's particular health history and develop a plan for how to ease symptoms.

Advance Directives

Advance directives are much more than a statement saying not to implement CPR or not to put someone on a ventilator. When done well, advance directives are a statement of someone's goals and values for healthcare at this time in her life. The goals can change over time, and so should the advance directive. These documents are effective only if they are part of the process of communicating with loved ones and healthcare providers.

An excellent tool for clarifying healthcare goals and values at any age is the material on the Prepare for Your Care website (Prepareforyourcare.org). If you or your loved one does not have an advance directive, please take a good look at that website. It features short videos and an easy-to-understand format to help clarify goals and values. It is an appropriate tool for people of all ages and in any state of health.

The advance directive forms on PrepareforYourCare.org are something that you and your loved one can complete without the help of a healthcare provider. These forms are legal in all fifty states. If you complete the forms, be sure to make copies of them and keep one copy at home, one copy at your doctor's office, and one copy that stays with your loved one.

Orders for Life-Sustaining Treatments (POLST)

Ask if your healthcare provider is familiar with the Physicians/Providers Order for Life-Sustaining Treatments (POLST) form. You can read more about it at POLST.org.

The POLST form is most appropriate for people with very serious, end-stage illness or those who are of very advanced age. You can complete this form with your doctor or advanced practice nurse (APN). The POLST form is likely to be more effective than many other advance directives or a living will because it is a legal medical order that specifies preferences. Also, since it involves your healthcare provider directly, she is part of the planning process.

In general, a living will or other advance directive is a paper that you completed, and your doctor or APN is not involved. The POLST form gives you and your loved one the opportunity to have an in-depth discussion with your healthcare provider and outline your priorities for care under certain circumstances. If you complete a POLST form, it is important to ensure that your doctor or APN signs it and that you each keep a copy of the form. However, before even exploring the idea of a POLST form, you need to clarify what the priorities are regarding healthcare decisions.

It is not necessary to have both a POLST form and another advance directive, such as one from the Prepare for Your Care website, but it is vital to have one or the other to make the best use of the suggestions in this book.

Medications

Make a list of all medications that your loved one takes. Include prescribed drugs as well as over-the-counter medications and supplements. Many people take acetaminophen, ibuprofen, or other medication on a regular basis, and your healthcare provider should be aware of all of them.

Vaccinations

Many national pharmacy chain stores give vaccinations, and they are covered by most health insurance plans.

Flu Vaccine: Every year, more than 30,000 people in the United States die from influenza. In just the first month of 2018, there were an average of 4,000 deaths each week from flu complications.

Older people and those with complex medical problems, such as cardiac disease, kidney failure, diabetes, lung/breathing problems, and dementia, are especially vulnerable to the devastating effects of the flu. In addition, those who are not vaccinated are more likely to spread the flu to other fragile people, such as small children and other family members.

You may have heard that the flu vaccine is not always effective, and that is true. Every year, the vaccine is formulated before the flu season begins, in anticipation of which flu strains are expected to be most common that year. It varies year to year, but generally, the vaccine reduces the risk of illness by 40% to 60%. However, even if the particular formulation is not 100% effective, there is evidence that those who have gotten the vaccine are less ill if they do contract the flu. The benefits of getting the flu vaccine far outweigh any risks for most people. And, because the vaccine is created with inactivated virus, it is impossible to get the flu from the vaccine.

Pneumonia Vaccines: Similar to the flu vaccine, the pneumonia vaccines can prevent serious illness and death for vulnerable people. A common cause of hospitalization and death for older people is pneumonia. If your goals include avoiding illness and suffering, in addition to preventing hospitalizations, getting the recommended vaccinations is a key part of the plan.

The pneumococcal vaccines can prevent life-threatening infections of the lungs, blood, and brain. These infections can be especially devastating for older people.

The pneumococcal vaccine is recommended for:

- People who are age sixty-five or older.
- People with a chronic condition, such as heart, lung (including asthma), liver, kidney, sickle cell disease or diabetes.
- People with cancer or a weakened immune system, including the HIV infection.
- People with a missing or damaged spleen.
- People with cerebrospinal fluid leaks or cochlear implants.
- People with chronic alcoholism or who smoke cigarettes.

Shingles Vaccine: Shingles (caused by the varicella-zoster virus) is a painful illness that can emerge in people—later in life—who have had chicken pox earlier in their lives. It causes a blistering rash, and it can take months to recover from it. Some people develop a chronic nerve pain that lasts years after the virus is no longer active.

The CDC recommends that everyone over age fifty get two doses of the RZV type vaccine, which is the preferred vaccine, or one dose of the ZVL type if age sixty or older, even if you have had shingles in the past.

Screening Tests

There are, literally, hundreds of tests and procedures that screen for all manner of disease. But, whether your healthcare provider recommends a screening test or not depends on many factors. Also, you and your loved one need to consider your healthcare goals before consenting to have a test done.

Anytime a test was recommended for my mother, Alma, we always asked, "What will we do with the results of this test?" For instance, when Alma was ninety-eight, she had a very irritated, scaly patch of skin on her neck. Keeping in mind her goal of limiting visits to the doctor, we tried many strategies at home to relieve the irritation. However, putting ointment on it, covering it with a bandage, and other comfort measures were ineffective at soothing the area. We went to a general surgeon's office for evaluation, and he suggested removing it in his office, using a local anesthetic to numb the area. Taking off the scaly patch would allow the skin underneath to heal. When the surgeon said that he could send the specimen to pathology to rule out cancer, we declined. At ninety-eight years old, my mother knew that she would not consent to any further treatment even if there was skin cancer, and so the test was unnecessary for her.

In general, the American Cancer Society advises that age, as well as overall health status, be considered when deciding about cancer screening. A healthy person at age eighty-five who does not have significant medical problems has a life expectancy of nearly ten more years, but an eighty-five-year-old with multiple severe medical problems may live less than three years. Given this variability, it is important to consider individual circumstances when deciding about screening tests.

It is natural to ask, "What can it hurt?" when given the opportunity to get screened for colon cancer, for instance. In reality, most screening tests come with an element of risk, which is increased for older patients, especially those with multiple medical problems. Testing can lead to interventions that may pose a burden and not extend the life of a frail, older person. These patients have a higher likelihood of experiencing a complication from screening and decreased chances that they would benefit from treatment should cancer be diagnosed. Yet, the reality is that people who are older and frail are more often referred for testing. Those least able to benefit are given a disproportionate amount of screening.

Many experts recommend that life expectancy, as well as overall health of a person, be considered in regards to what cancer screenings should be performed.
After all, if your loved one has
a reasonable chance of living for five more years in relative peace, would you want to subject her to aggressive cancer biopsies and treatments that have serious side effects, if her other health problems (such as dementia, heart failure or emphysema) will limit her life, anyway? These other health problems will make her more susceptible to complications from aggressive testing and treatments.

Some Common Screening Tests and Considerations

1. Mammogram, for breast cancer: Women fifty-five and older should switch to mammograms every two years or can continue yearly screening. The American Cancer Society recommends that screening should continue as long as a woman is in good health and is expected to live ten more years or longer.

Risks of screening: Pain, anxiety and false positives leading to unnecessary further testing or surgery. Women diagnosed with breast cancer at an older age, especially those with other serious health problems, such as dementia, are more likely to die of something other than cancer. Therefore, screening older, sicker women may lead to more treatments that cause a burden without extending their lives.

2. Colonoscopy: According to the American Academy of Family Practice Physicians, routine screening in people ages seventy-six up to age eighty-five is not recommended, unless there is a specific rationale. For those over age eighty-five, screening is not recommended at all. The American Geriatrics Society also recommends not screening people who have a life expectancy of fewer than ten years, because the burdens of testing and treatments outweigh the small chance of benefits.

Risks of screening: Complications from sedation, colon perforation, adverse effects on the heart or lungs and bleeding. Risks increase for people with serious health problems, and the benefits of screening are fewer.

3. PSA for prostate cancer: The American Urological Association recommends that screening is not done for men older than seventy or with a life expectancy of less than ten to fifteen years.

Risks of screening: Over-diagnosis of prostate cancer increases with people over age seventy-four. If the PSA level is high, many patients will then have a biopsy, which has a high risk of pain, fever, bleeding, infection, urinary incontinence, or erectile dysfunction.

4. PAP smear, for cervical cancer: The American Cancer Society and the American College of Obstetricians and Gynecologists state that screening should not continue after age sixty-five in women who have had negative screenings in the prior five to ten years; the guidelines should be discussed with the doctor before screening, especially for women who have had a hysterectomy.

Risks of screening: Pain and discomfort, false positives that may lead to additional procedures and biopsies.

Appendix 4

Renal Failure and Dialysis

Kidney disease is common in the United States among older adults, affecting more than 30% of people over the age of sixty-five. Diabetes and high blood pressure are two of the contributing causes of kidney problems, and both of these chronic conditions need to be well controlled to lessen the risks of permanent kidney damage.

The unfortunate truth is that many people with early stages of kidney damage are unaware of it. It is in the early stages that modifications in diet and medications have the best chance to reduce the effects and progression of the disease. If you are helping an older loved one with medical issues, it is a good idea to ask his healthcare provider if there is any kidney damage and what can be done to stop it from progressing.

When kidney disease does progress to kidney failure, often after a severe illness such as a heart attack or a serious infection, dialysis may be needed. Kidney failure (also called End Stage Renal Disease, or ESRD) is an enormous problem in the United States. More than 650,000 people deal with the effects of this disease every year. Most receive dialysis, and many live with the hope of receiving a kidney transplant. For the vast majority of people, a transplant will not be an option, so dialysis is the only alternative.

Starting dialysis involves having a catheter inserted that allows for access to the vein and artery needed to dialyze the blood. Most people then have an operation to have an arterial-venous fistula created in the arm. This fistula is considered safer for dialysis and has fewer risks of complications from infections. The fistula is under the skin and creates a connection between an artery and vein in the arm. It is where the dialysis nurse will connect the patient to the dialysis machine.

Another form of dialysis is peritoneal dialysis. This is usually done at home every day as opposed to hemo-dialysis, which is done at a dialysis center several times a week.

Five years is the average life expectancy for someone who is over sixty-five years old and on dialysis. For those who are over age seventy-five when they start dialysis, more than 80% die within the first five years. These facts are grim, and yet, most people on dialysis are not aware that their life expectancy is so short.

Studies show that people with kidney failure want to know the severity of their disease and the facts about their life expectancy. Yet, more than 90% say they have not discussed it with their doctors. This lack of communication about their prognosis robs patients of the ability to make informed decisions and lessens the chances that their goals and values will be the driving force in their care. While dialysis can be lifesaving, it comes at a great cost for an older, frail person. It is important to know the facts so that you can make informed decisions about whether to start or to continue dialysis.

Here are some key facts:

- Most ESRD patients have dialysis three times a week, and it takes approximately four hours each time.

- Within the first year of dialysis, 40% of people older than age seventy-five will die.

- People on dialysis have a high rate of hospitalizations and high-cost care at the end of life.

- People who are frail when they start dialysis generally become more frail and dependent.

- Many dialysis patients report that their chronic pain that is not very well-controlled by medication.

- Nursing home patients who start dialysis have a significant decline in physical and mental functioning within three months of starting dialysis.

Questions to Ask Regarding Dialysis:

1. What is the realistic prognosis/life expectancy with this diagnosis?

2. How do my other medical problems affect the prognosis?

3. Will dialysis improve my quality of life?

4. Are there other ways to manage kidney disease, instead of dialysis?

5. Can you refer us to a palliative-care provider who will help manage the side effects of dialysis and kidney disease?

6. What problems are common in the first year of dialysis?

Being on dialysis is a big adjustment for patients and their families. Many people report that they started dialysis not knowing the limited life expectancy and that they felt pressured into the treatment. ESRD is a terminal diagnosis that has to be understood in order to make informed decisions. It is important to clarify the goals and values regarding health-care during this vulnerable time. An older person on dialysis is near the end of her life, meaning that the vast majority of dialysis patients will not live longer than three to five years. Take advantage of that information to have the important, planning conversations with your loved ones.

A good understanding of the goals and values will help you to be in control of the healthcare process rather than being on the conveyor belt.

Appendix 5

Medications that are Potentially Harmful to Older Patients

Experts have identified high-risk medications that require great caution for use in older people. If your loved one is prescribed one of these medications, it is reasonable to ask her healthcare professional if a safer alternative is available. Always use medications as prescribed, and never discontinue a medication without speaking to the appropriate physician.

Please refer to the chart on the following page.

Antihistamines:	Heart Medication:	Barbiturates:	Pain Medication:	Nausea:
diphenhydramine (Benedryl)	disopyramide (Norpace, Norpace CR)	amobarbital (Amytal)	meperidine (Demerol)	trimethobenzamide (Tigan)
brompheniramine	digoxin (dose of more than 0.125 mg/day) (Lanoxin)	butabarbital (Butisol)	pentazocine (Talacen, Talwin)	Oral Medication for Diabetes:
carbinoxamine	nifedipine (immediate-release)	butalbital (Fioricet, Fiorinal)	Pain Medication NSAIDS:	chlorpropamide (Diabinese)
chlorpheniramine	Blood Pressure:	pentobarbital (Nembutal)	indomethacin (Indocin)	glyburide (Diabeta, Glynase, Micronase)
clemastine	guanfacine (Tenex)	phenobarbital (Liminal)	ketorolac (Sprix, Toradol)	Benzodiazipine/ Sedatives:
cyproheptadine (Periactin)	methyldopa (Aldomet)	secobarbital (Seconal)	Muscle Relaxants:	diazepam (Valium)
dexbrompheniramine	reserpine (more than 0.1 mg/day)	Sedative/ Hypnotic	carisoprodol (SOMA)	lorazepam (Ativan)
dexchlorpheniramine	guanfacine (Intuniv)	chloral hydrate (Somnote)	chlorzoxazone (Lorsone, Parafon Forte DSC)	alprazolam (Xanax)
doxylamine	Antidepressants	meprobamate (Miltown)	cyclobenzaprine (Flexeril)	chlordiazepoxide (Librium)
hydroxyzine (Atarax, Vistaril)	amitriptyline (Elavil)	Other Hypnotics:	metaxalone (Skelaxin)	flurazepam (Dalmane)
promethazine (Phenergan)	amitriptyline/chlordiazepoxide (Limbitrol)	eszopiclone (Lunesta)	methocarbamol (Robaxin)	Anti-Psychotic:
triprolidine	amitriptyline/perphenazine (Triavil)	zolpidem (Ambien)	orphenadrine (Norflex)	thioridazine (Mellaril)
Parkinson's Disease Medications:	clomipramine (Anafranil)	zaleplon (Sonata)	Antibiotic:	Drugs Affecting Blood Clotting:
benztropine oral (Cogentin)	doxepin (more than 6 mg/day) (Sinequan)	Vasodilators for dementia:	levofloxacin (Levaquin)	dipyridamole (Persantine)
trihexyphenidyl (Artane)	imipramine (Tofranil, Tofranil-PM)	ergoloid mesylates (Hydergine)	nitrofurantoin (Macrobid, Macrodantin)	ticlopidine (Ticlid)
	trimipramine (Surmontil)	isoxsuprine (Vasodilan)		

Appendix 6

A Summary of Key Points

Setting Goals

Setting healthcare and lifestyle goals are essential to having a clear plan when things go wrong. Once an illness strikes, emotions and fear often take over. You may find yourself with your loved one in the emergency room, uncomfortable and upset. At that point, it is difficult to think clearly. Before you know it, you are on the healthcare conveyor belt, and you do not know how to get off.

Recommended resources to explore:

1. PrepareForYourCare.org

2. TheConversationProject.org

3. AARP.org

Frailty

Having the responsibility of helping another person with healthcare decisions can be overwhelming. It can be difficult to know what to recommend when faced with questions about preventative care, such as cancer screenings or a proposed surgery. An important fact to keep in mind is that not all older people are alike. There are many differences among people who reach the age of seventy-six, for instance.

At that age, Alma was living independently, driving every day, had an active social life, and had no chronic medical problems. She lived twenty-three more years in good health. Compare that to Janet from Chapter 6. Janet was seventy-six, but lived in a nursing home; having advanced dementia, she no longer recognized her family. Two prior strokes left her bedridden, and severe COPD caused her difficulty with breathing. Janet's medical history made her quite frail and vulnerable to many complications from any medical intervention. An estimated 40% of the people with Janet's health problems die within six months, and virtually all die within ten years. If Janet's family had known the impact that her frail condition had on her life expectancy, they might have made different healthcare choices for her.

Frailty is an important component to consider when making healthcare decisions. Healthcare specialists use many different ways to calculate a patient's frailty. Most calculations consider:

- The number of chronic medical problems—of particular concern for increased frailty are heart failure, COPD, kidney disease, cancer and dementia.

- How much help the person needs to accomplish simple self-care tasks, such as eating, toileting and dressing.

- Can the person walk?

- Has there been a recent weight loss?

Frailty is a vulnerability to physical stress, such as sudden illness and the stress caused by chronic long-term conditions. If your loved one has many of these characteristics, it may be an important element to bring up in your discussions with healthcare providers.

Informed Consent

Even when the informed-consent process is done strictly "by the book," it is not enough. Instead of presenting the patient and family with a form to sign and a canned speech about risks and benefits, we should start with a conversation about goals. This is especially important for patients who are frail, dealing with multiple medical problems or who are older. We have to ask what the patient hopes to achieve from the surgery. It is important to know if the surgery will help her to accomplish her goals.

It is important to remember that even someone with a diagnosis of dementia may have the capacity to give consent for treatments, tests, and surgeries. Giving a careful explanation, done in a way that gives the older person time to process what is being said as well as time to ask questions, is key.

Going to the Hospital

For frail, older people, being in the hospital can present a minefield of danger. Not only are they subject to risks of infection and increased confusion, but also the treatment they receive can seem inhumane. While each patient is unique, there are some commonly occurring adverse events for older people in the hospital. Being aware of these risks may help you to advocate for your loved one and avoid hospitalization, or take steps to mitigate the risks while in the hospital.

Older patients, especially those with any level of dementia or with multiple medical problems are at risk for developing delirium while in the hospital. Up to 87% of patients older than the age of sixty-five will have episodes of delirium while in the ICU.

Will the Burden Outweigh the Benefit?

There are always more tests that can be done. Will the burden outweigh the benefit? Any time a procedure, test or medication is recommended, be sure to ask if the likely benefits will be greater than the burdens that may be brought to your loved one by the intervention. Many tests, medications, and procedures pose more risks than benefits for older people.

Feeding Tubes

The American Society of Geriatrics specifically recommends that people with advanced dementia do not get feeding tubes because the evidence shows it is not a benefit to them and that tube-feedings cause real harm. These doctors who specialize in the care of patients over age sixty-five point out that pneumonia, febrile episodes, and eating problems represent a natural progression of the disease process and indicate a transition from advanced dementia to end of life.

Palliative Care: A Better Way

Palliative care is a specialty in medicine that focuses on treating the distressing symptoms of serious illness. It is appropriate to have palliative care at any stage of a serious illness. The goals for palliative care include not only treating the physical symptoms that cause suffering but also helping patients and families deal with the stress of serious or chronic illness and in assisting the patient to live his best possible life.

Patients who have the benefit of palliative care experience less depression and even live longer than patients who received exclusively traditional care. Family members of palliative-care patients receive a benefit as well, experiencing less stress, anxiety, and depression.

Caregiver Care

While it is true that you cannot help someone else as effectively when you are worn out and overwhelmed, finding the time to take care of yourself can also be difficult. Sometimes a change of attitude is helpful. When I have found myself at the end of my rope while caring for a loved one, I realize that what was most frustrating me was the feeling of being out of control. It is tempting to feel that you want to make things better and that if everyone just acted according to your plan, life would be easier. But, it does not work that way. Being responsible for another adult's most personal matters brings a tangle of emotions and complications on all sides. Do not neglect yourself during these stressful times.

Resources

I have a useful list of resources that will help you to learn more about the topics covered in this book. Because I am always learning of new resources and people who can help you, it makes sense to put the list online in order to keep it updated. Please go to *GettingTheBestCare.com* to see the resources section, it is free and you do not need to register.

Notes on Sources

I read countless research studies and journal articles while preparing to write this book. If I listed them all here it would have made the book at least 20 pages longer-and that means more expensive! So, I decided to put the Notes on Sources section online. On the website *GettingTheBestCare.com*, you can see all of the articles and studies that I used organized according to book chapter.

> *But to expose the former faults of any person, without knowing what their present feelings were, seems unjustifiable.*
> —Jane Bennet in *Pride and Prejudice*, by Jane Austin

Regarding the use of Pronouns

One legacy that my mother left to her children was a respect for proper grammar. I cannot pretend to be the expert that she was regarding proper sentence structure, but I am ever-hopeful of improvement. One development I have observed in recent years is the increasing use of plural pronouns (them, they, their) in sentences with a singular antecedent as in: The patient asked their doctor about the medication. This is the sort of grammar faux pas that Alma would find distracting, to say the least.

However, I have learned in the writing, and editing process of this book, that using "their, them or they" as gender non-specific pronouns is now an accepted option. The Merriam-Webster dictionary affirms its use to refer to an individual person whose "gender is not known or specified." And this issue has taken on increased significance for a society that seeks to include all people. I am sorry to admit that I was unaware of this evolution in grammar when I wrote the manuscript for this book—although, apparently, Jane Austen was on board over two hundred years ago. I am hopeful that readers of all persuasions will understand that this book and its content is meant for them.

Acknowledgments

Regarding this book, as with many things in my life, it is most appropriate to thank my mother, Alma. Her grace in aging, and tenacity in living life with autonomy is a source of inspiration for this book and my work in general, as well as for my life.

Professionally, I have been fortunate to have had many mentors. As a new graduate nurse, I was privileged to work under Dr. Charles von Gunten and Dr. Kathy J. Neely at Northwestern Memorial Hospital in Chicago. Their work on the Hospice and Palliative Care Unit taught me so much about what it means to provide compassionate and intelligent care to patients. Drs. Ira Byock and Atul Gawande have been inspirations to me even though I have never met them. Through their writings they have helped to educate the public as well as healthcare professionals about giving individualized care that respects patient's values.

In the making of this book I am grateful for the work of Dave Chilton (author of *The Wealthy Barber*) who so generously shares his expertise in writing, publishing and marketing. Kristen Havens, Andrea Cumbo-Floyd, Yvonne Mullins and Samantha Paquin provided editing expertise without which, this book would be unreadable! Thank you, also to

Christy Collins for her artistic cover design and to Nick Zelinger, for the interior design.

Most of all, there is my husband Jim. The kindest and most generous person I know, without his support and encouragement I could not have completed this project. His faith in me is both humbling and a source of fuel which pushes me forward. LUM.

About the Author

Margaret Fitzpatrick has over twenty years of experience in critical care nursing; first as an ICU and Trauma Nurse Specialist and now as a Nurse Anesthetist. She received her Master's degree in Science from Rosalind Franklin University of Medicine and Science. Margaret has spent her career as a Nurse Anesthetist in community hospitals serving primarily inner-city populations in and around Chicago.

Coming from a large family with 15 siblings, Margaret has had years of experience helping many family members and friends navigate the healthcare system at all stages of life. She is dedicated to empowering patients and their family members with the knowledge that the best medical care is based on individualized goals set by the patient. Her prior book, *What to Ask the Doc: The Questions to Ask to Get the Answers You Need*, published in 2003 by RN Interactive Publishing, was co-authored by Linda (Burke) Louis, R.N., and Daryl Lee, R.N.

Margaret and her husband, Jim McLaughlin, live south of Chicago, sharing the home of their benevolent border collie, Betty.

Quantity Discounts are available.

At certain quantities the author will make presentations to your organization, school or business.

For details please contact:
Margaret@GettingTheBestCare.com

Video of the author is at:
GettingTheBestCare.com

Index